Parkinson's Disease

A PERSONAL ACCOUNT IN PICTURES
BY TERRY RUMMINS

Illustrations by Jack Rummins

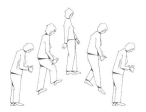

9 39830416

Copyright © 2013 Terry Rummins

The moral right of the author has been asserted.

Apart from any fair dealing for the purposes of research or private study,
or criticism or review, as permitted under the Copyright, Designs and Patents
Act 1988, this publication may only be reproduced, stored or transmitted, in
any form or by any means, with the prior permission in writing of the
publishers, or in the case of reprographic reproduction in accordance with
the terms of licences issued by the Copyright Licensing Agency. Enquiries
concerning reproduction outside those terms should be sent to the publishers.

Matador
9 Priory Business Park
Kibworth Beauchamp
Leicestershire LE8 0RX, UK
Tel: (+44) 116 279 2299
Fax: (+44) 116 279 2277
Email: books@troubador.co.uk
Web: www.troubador.co.uk/matador

ISBN 978 1780885 520

British Library Cataloguing in Publication Data.
A catalogue record for this book is available from the British Library.

Matador is an imprint of Troubador Publishing Ltd

To anybody who is living with Parkinson's Disease.

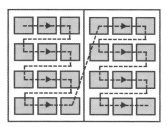

Read each page from left to right.
The story and graphic panels are sequential.

downwards, 'never' becoming a
reality, in slow motion. Every
time I have become aware of
some other ability that I am los-
... ing I have
... felt that I
... am wit-
nessing
... my own
... slow
... death, my
... own de-
... construc-
tion. At
... those
times I worr... out the future.
What will he... if I can't manage to look a... elf at all?
Am I bec...
ever the p...
the other...
chance oc...
encourage...
ple of the...
one asks...
advice. A...
is when I...
'achievem...
started a v...
have man...
over the p...
my recent...
maintainin...
and devel...
to live for...
fairly rea...
life in En...
at a time,...
by taking...
sations an...
books, ge...
widely th...
learning t...

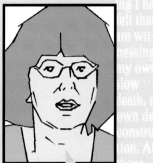

ONCE UPON
A TIME.....

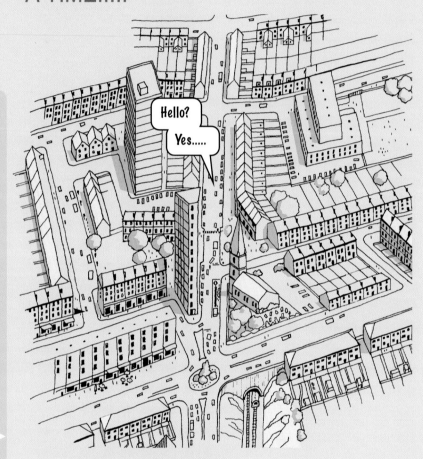

Hello?

Yes.....

Hello, I'm Terry
In response to a minor tremor
that had started in my right
hand, I was diagnosed as having
Parkinson's Disease. However, it
seems likely that I began
developing the condition much
earlier.
At the time of diagnosis I was
fifty-eight years old, working
full-time, married and with a
family. The diagnosis was a
shock and it conjured up all
sorts of fears in my mind, but I
had no idea what having
Parkinson's meant in reality.
Well, ten years on, this story,
describes what it has meant
to me....

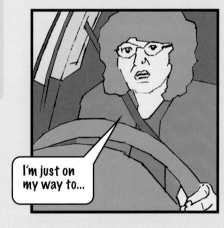

I'm just on
my way to...

I HAD A
BUSY
WORKING
LIFE....

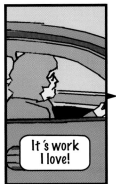

It's work I love!

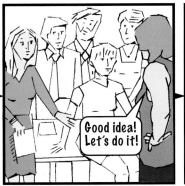

Good idea! Let's do it!

Hello, I'm Terry. Please take a seat.

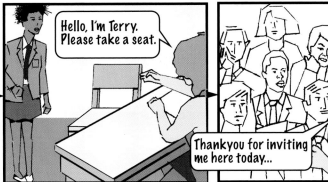

Thankyou for inviting me here today...

THEN

MY RIGHT HAND STARTED SHAKING

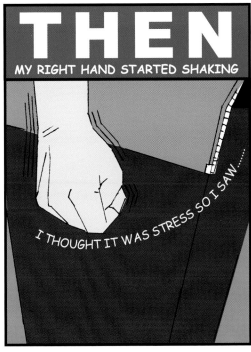

I THOUGHT IT WAS STRESS SO I SAW.......

......MY GP

A HYPNO-THERAPIST

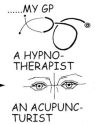

AN ACUPUNC-TURIST

AND A HOMEOPATH

BUT THE TREMOR CONTINUED AND...

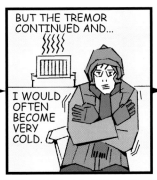

I WOULD OFTEN BECOME VERY COLD.

ALSO, MY WRITING GOT SMALLER

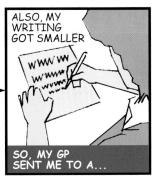

SO, MY GP SENT ME TO A...

CONSULTANT NEUROLOGIST

WHO ASKED ME TO WRITE:

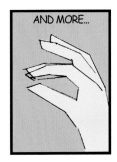

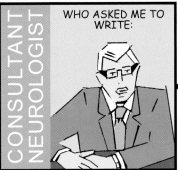

Mary had a little lamb
Mary had a little lamb
Mary had a little lamb
Mary had a little lamb
Mary had a little lamb
Mary had a little lamb

NEXT, TO TAP MY ...	FINGER & THUMB.	THIS BECAME...	MORE...	AND MORE...	DIFFICULT.

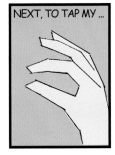 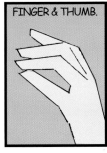 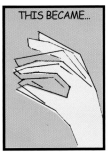 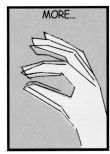 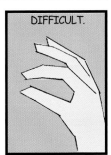

AND THEN TO

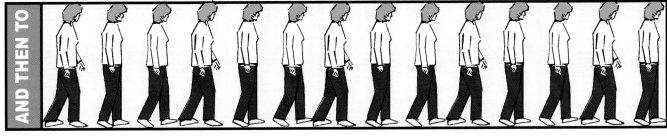

MY HUSBAND, JACK, WHO HAD ACCOMPANIED ME, NOTICED THE LACK OF MOVEMENT IN MY RIGHT ARM AS I WALKED UP AND DOWN...

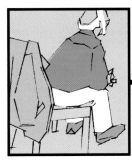

THE CONSULTANT THEN PLACED HIS HANDS ON MY SHOULDERS...

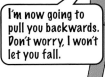

I'm now going to pull you backwards. Don't worry, I won't let you fall.

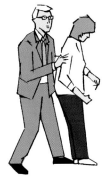

and finally he said.........

2

"You have Parkinson's Disease, a degenerative neurological condition which will never improve, will steadily get worse and for which there is no cure."

I DIDN'T KNOW **WHAT TO FEEL.**

I IMAGINED ALL SORTS OF FUTURES FOR MYSELF. I EVEN IMAGINED THAT IT WAS ALL A BIG MISTAKE...

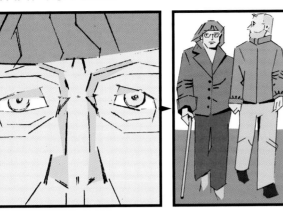
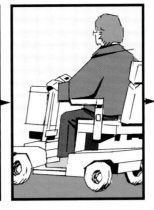
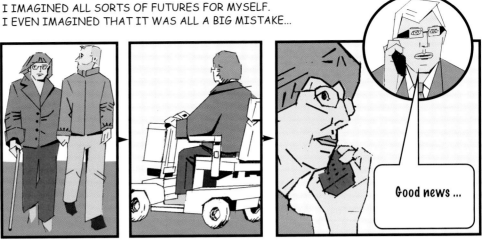

Good news ...

I WONDERED WHAT **OTHER PEOPLE** WOULD THINK OF ME.

I OFTEN ADDRESS LARGE GROUPS OF PEOPLE....

Daily activities became...

more and more of a struggle...

leading to exhaustion and...

feelings of frustration.

You may notice that I'm shaking...

Terry, I'm so sorry to hear that you have Parkinson's....

But it's awful...

That's good Terry, but....

OH, I THINK IT IS!

I talked openly about my disability:

How long have you had it, Terry?

About two years, I think.

Is it painful?

Some people have pain, but thankfully I don't.

I tried to understand why some people didn't want me to be positive....

Thankyou. Fortunately there are good drugs....

There's also a lot of research...

At least it's not life threatening....

I discovered the usefulness of imperfection;

Why you shaking Miss?

Oh...my gran's got that. She gets stuck doin' things. D'you get that, Miss?

I've got Parkinson's disease.

and tried to avoid ascribing negative thoughts to others.

She thinks I can't do my job.

She must find it difficult...

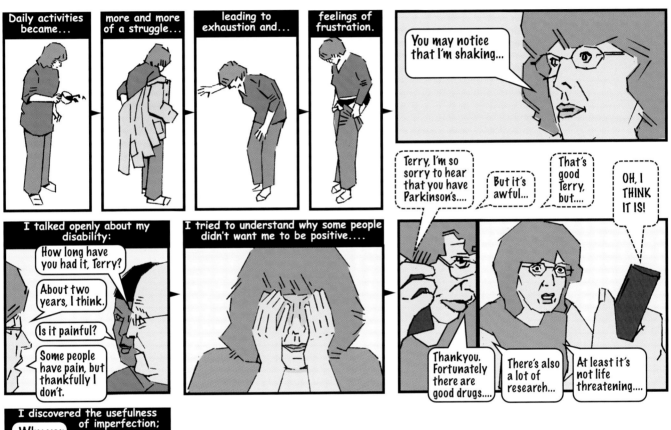
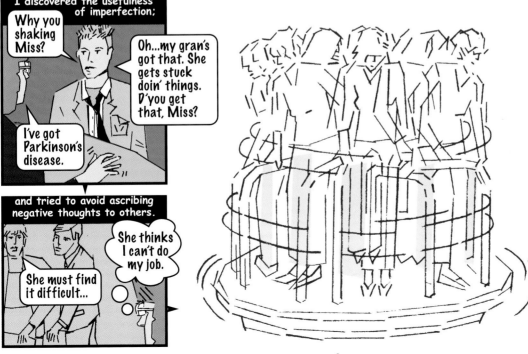

AS I BECAME MORE UNWELL I COULD SEE THAT REALITY WAS CHANGING FOR ME. MY OPTIONS WERE UNCLEAR. I WOULD HAVE TO BUILD A NEW UNDERSTANDING OF MYSELF.

FIRST OF ALL, I NEEDED TO KNOW
WHAT I WAS UP AGAINST. SO....

THIS WAY I RECEIVED SOME THEORY;
I LEARNED ABOUT SYMPTOMS...

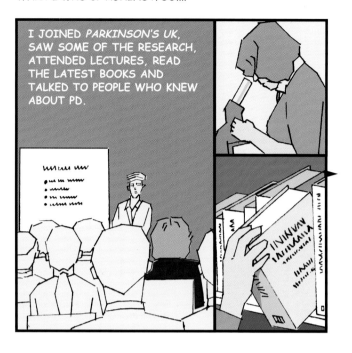

I JOINED *PARKINSON'S UK*,
SAW SOME OF THE RESEARCH,
ATTENDED LECTURES, READ
THE LATEST BOOKS AND
TALKED TO PEOPLE WHO KNEW
ABOUT PD.

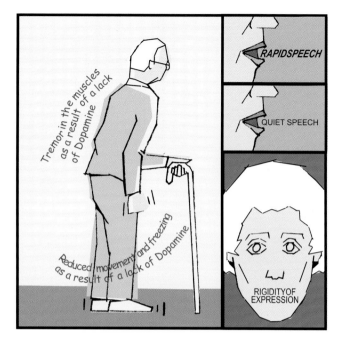

Tremor in the muscles as a result of a lack of Dopamine

Reduced movement and freezing as a result of a lack of Dopamine

RAPID SPEECH

QUIET SPEECH

RIGIDITY OF EXPRESSION

AND MEDICATION....

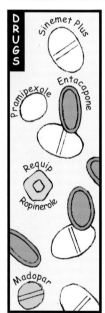

Sinemet Plus includes
Levodopa (which is
converted into
Dopamine in the body).

Pramipexole is a
Dopamine Agonist that
imitates the effects
of Dopamine.

Entacapone slows
the breakdown of
Levodopa in the body.

Ropinerole is a
Dopamine Agonist that
imitates the effects
of Dopamine.

Madopar includes
Levodopa (which is
converted into
Dopamine in the body).

I ALSO DISCOVERED THAT NO ONE KNOWS THE CAUSE OF PARKINSON'S.
GENERALLY SPEAKING, IT SEEMS TO OCCUR AS THE RESULT OF INTERACTION
BETWEEN ENVIRONMENTAL FACTORS (SUCH AS THE USE OF PESTICIDES), AND
UNKNOWN GENETIC TENDENCIES THAT ....

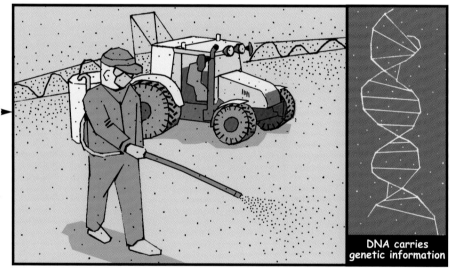

DNA carries
genetic information

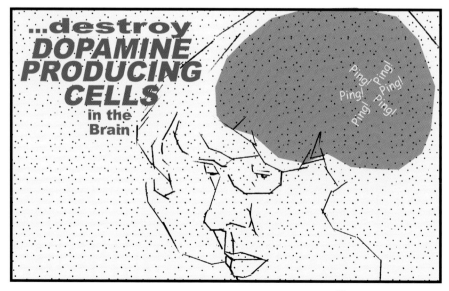

...destroy
DOPAMINE
PRODUCING
CELLS
in the
Brain

Ping! Ping!
Ping! Ping!
Ping! Ping!

"I remember as a
young girl, in Malta,
walking to school
through areas that
were regularly
sprayed with
chemicals to kill
insects."

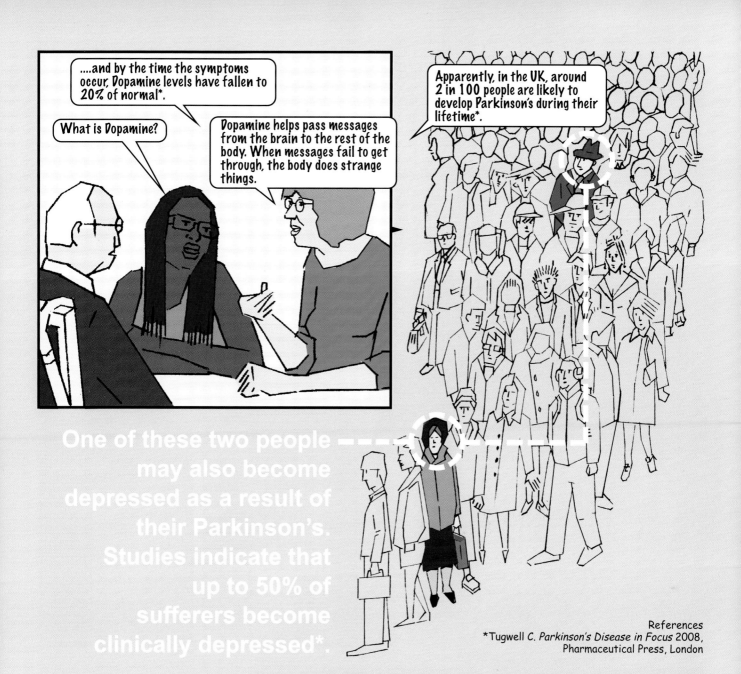

One of these two people may also become depressed as a result of their Parkinson's. Studies indicate that up to 50% of sufferers become clinically depressed*.

References
*Tugwell C. *Parkinson's Disease in Focus* 2008, Pharmaceutical Press, London

MORE MEN THAN WOMEN DEVELOP PARKINSON'S. ITS PROGRESS DIFFERS FROM PERSON TO PERSON AND MAY BE INFLUENCED BY: GENERAL HEALTH; ATTITUDE; PERSONALITY; AND RESPONSE TO MEDICATION.

Shortly after diagnosis my medication was 1mg of 'Ropinerole' five times a day prescribed by my consultant and a 40mg Beta blocker a day prescribed by my GP for tremor. A year later, I was taking 2mg of 'Ropinerole' five times a day, plus the Beta blocker. I was told that Dopamine agonists, such as 'Ropinerole' are generally not as effective as 'Sinemet' or 'Madopar' which convert levodopa into Dopamine, but they have the advantage that they are less likely to lead to dyskinesias which become evident after long-term usage of levodopa.

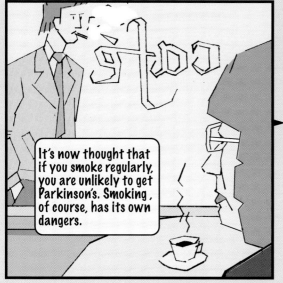

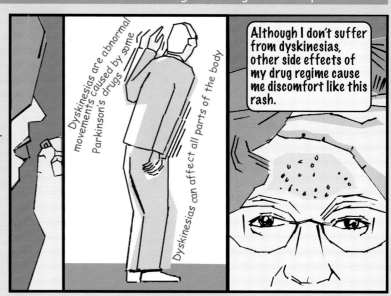

THE MOST IMPORTANT LESSON I LEARNED WAS TO ABANDON PHYSICAL EFFORT AND PERSEVERENCE TO GET THINGS DONE. THIS ONCE SUCCESSFUL TECHNIQUE NOW LEAVES ME EXHAUSTED, DISPIRITED AND DESPERATE.

Parkinson's has no respect for effort or repetition.

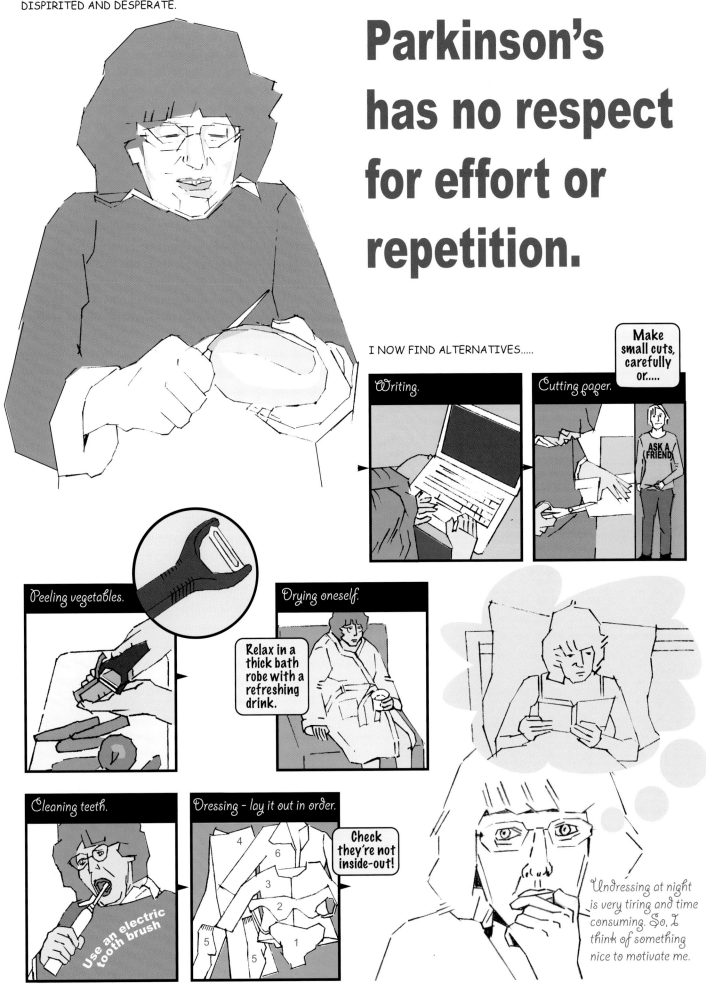

I NOW FIND ALTERNATIVES.....

Writing.

Cutting paper.

Make small cuts, carefully or.....

ASK A FRIEND

Peeling vegetables.

Drying oneself.

Relax in a thick bath robe with a refreshing drink.

Cleaning teeth.

Use an electric tooth brush

Dressing - lay it out in order.

Check they're not inside-out!

Undressing at night is very tiring and time consuming. So, I think of something nice to motivate me.

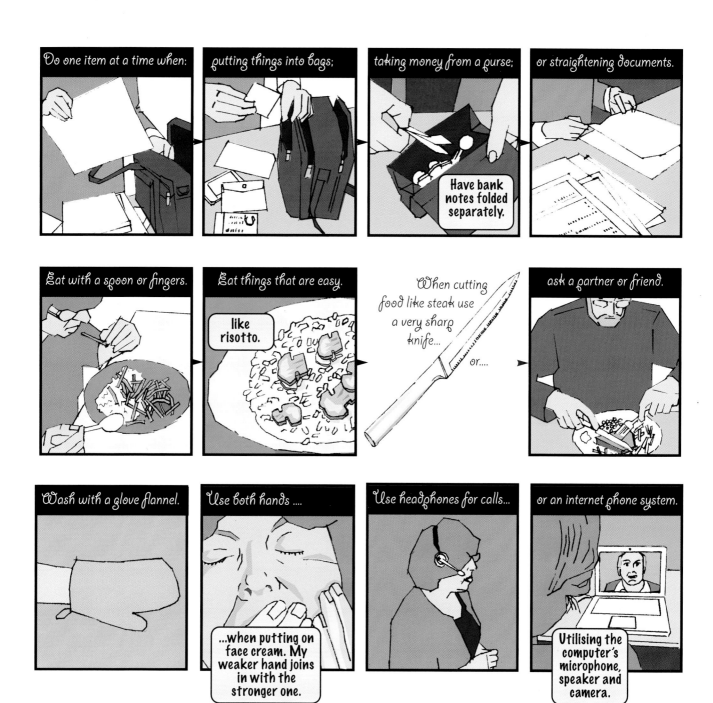

Do one item at a time when:

putting things into bags;

taking money from a purse;

Have bank notes folded separately.

or straightening documents.

Eat with a spoon or fingers.

Eat things that are easy.

like risotto.

When cutting food like steak use a very sharp knife... or....

ask a partner or friend.

Wash with a glove flannel.

Use both hands ....

...when putting on face cream. My weaker hand joins in with the stronger one.

Use headphones for calls...

or an internet phone system.

Utilising the computer's microphone, speaker and camera.

MY MOST SPECTACULAR SUCCESS IS FINDING A WAY TO GET UP FROM A LOW CHAIR OR THE BATH....

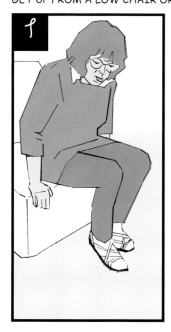

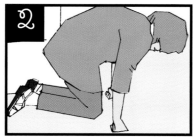

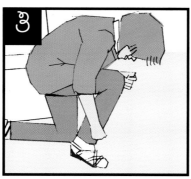

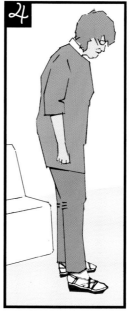

Sometimes, when I become very tired, muscles in my right arm and back tighten up and hurt. Then, I just feel like keeping still and letting the world go by.

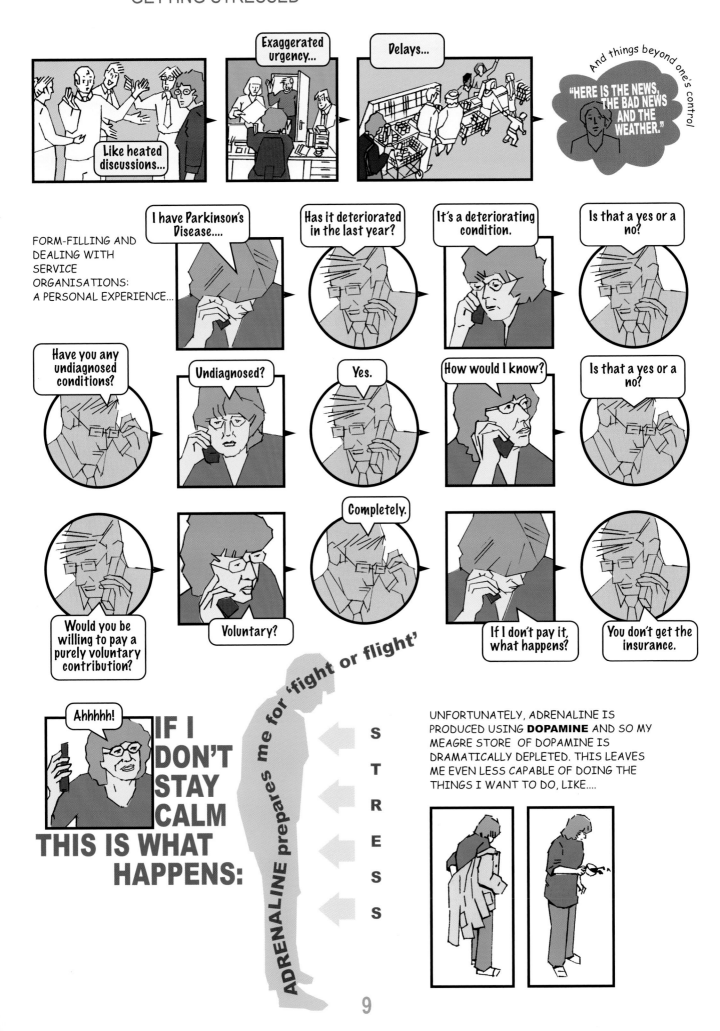

PRACTISE RELAXATION TECHNIQUES...

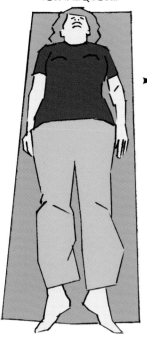

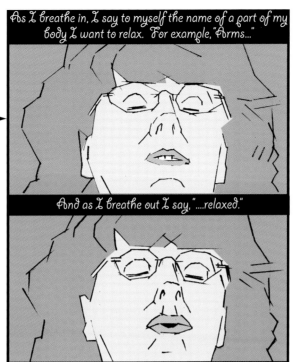

As I breathe in, I say to myself the name of a part of my body I want to relax. For example, "Arms..."

And as I breathe out I say, "....relaxed."

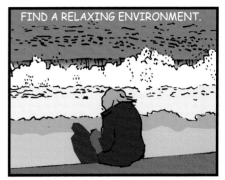

FIND A RELAXING ENVIRONMENT.

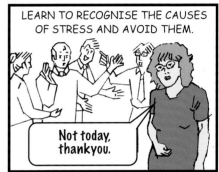

LEARN TO RECOGNISE THE CAUSES OF STRESS AND AVOID THEM.

Not today, thankyou.

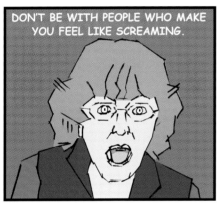

DON'T BE WITH PEOPLE WHO MAKE YOU FEEL LIKE SCREAMING.

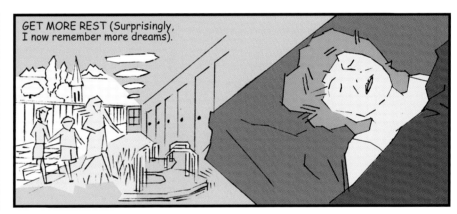

GET MORE REST (Surprisingly, I now remember more dreams).

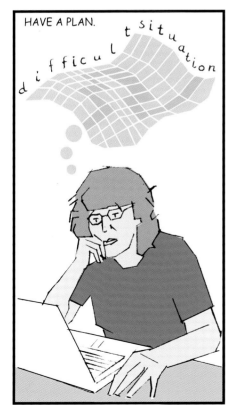

HAVE A PLAN.

difficult situation

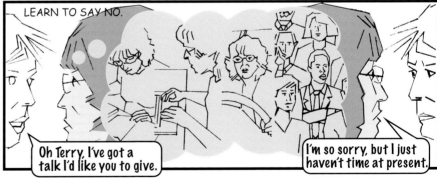

LEARN TO SAY NO.

Oh Terry, I've got a talk I'd like you to give.

I'm so sorry, but I just haven't time at present.

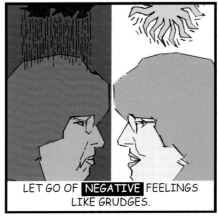

LET GO OF NEGATIVE FEELINGS LIKE GRUDGES.

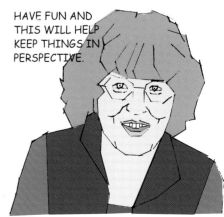

HAVE FUN AND THIS WILL HELP KEEP THINGS IN PERSPECTIVE.

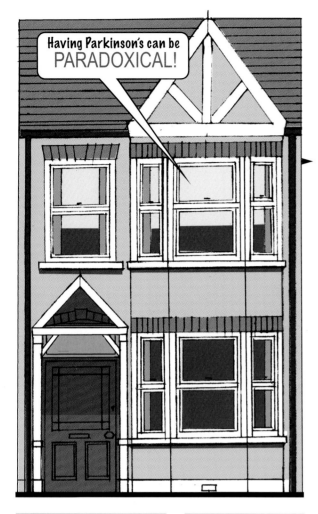

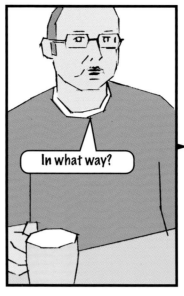

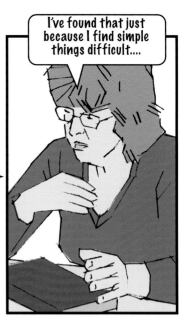

LIKE....　　　AND....　　　AND WALKING IN A STRAIGHT LINE....

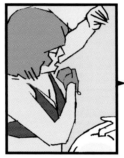

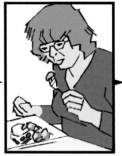

LIKE GIVING TALKS...　　AND COMPOSING DETAILED REPORTS.

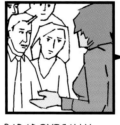

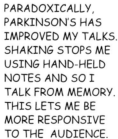

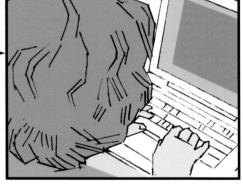

PARADOXICALLY, PARKINSON'S HAS IMPROVED MY TALKS. SHAKING STOPS ME USING HAND-HELD NOTES AND SO I TALK FROM MEMORY. THIS LETS ME BE MORE RESPONSIVE TO THE AUDIENCE.

IN TYPING REPORTS I EXPECTED MY RIGHT HAND TO TIRE QUICKLY AND TYPE MORE AND MORE SLOWLY. BUT IT FOLLOWED MY LEFT HAND AND MOVED FASTER THAN I EXPECTED.

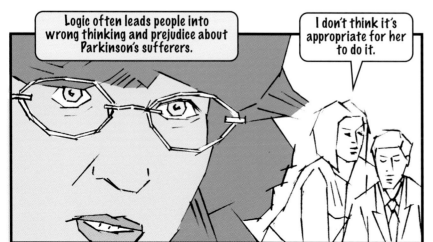

With Parkinson's, assumptions are a waste of time.

IMAGINATION IS WHAT IS NEEDED!

THE DRUG THAT I HAVE FOUND INVALUABLE IN HELPING MY SYMPTOMS OF PARKINSON'S IS LEVODOPA (SINEMET PLUS) WHICH I STARTED TAKING FIVE YEARS AFTER DIAGNOSIS. BEFORE THAT I HAD BEEN TAKING 'ROPINEROLE'.

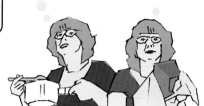

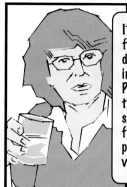

I've been taking 'Ropinerole' for five years, following my diagnosis, and it's proved ineffective against my Parkinson's. Side effects of the drug; dry mouth and sleepiness, have affected me from the start. Sleepiness, particularly, has become very stressful.

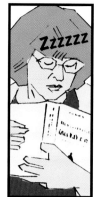

Zzzzzz

But what is surprising is an increase in my sex-drive.

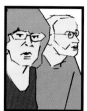

In the future Jack will look back to this period with amused nostalgia.

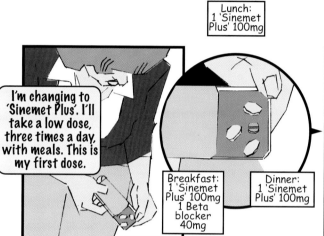

I'm changing to 'Sinemet Plus'. I'll take a low dose, three times a day, with meals. This is my first dose.

Lunch:
1 'Sinemet Plus' 100mg

Breakfast:
1 'Sinemet Plus' 100mg
1 Beta blocker 40mg

Dinner:
1 'Sinemet Plus' 100mg

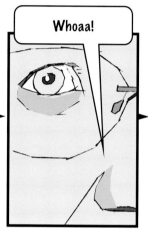

Whoaa!

HOT
SWEATY
FAINT

The side effects are horrible. So, I decrease the dose to half a tablet, three times a day, with meals.

This provides only a small improvement. I'm having to arrange my work around my drugs.

Then, I found that in some people, protein and Levodopa compete to cross the blood-brain barrier and the result is that those people are physically upset.

I am one of those people and I feel like a battleground.

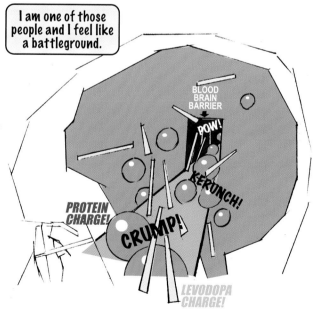

BLOOD BRAIN BARRIER

POW!

KERUNCH!

CRUMP!

PROTEIN CHARGE!

LEVODOPA CHARGE!

SO, NEARLY SIX YEARS AFTER DIAGNOSIS, I STOPPED EATING PROTEIN WITH BREAKFAST AND LUNCH AND TOOK MY HALF TABLET OF SINEMET PLUS (LEVODOPA) AT LEAST AN HOUR AND A QUARTER BEFORE EACH OF THESE MEALS. I TOOK MY THIRD HALF TABLET JUST BEFORE GOING TO BED, ALLOWING ME TO HAVE PROTEIN WITH DINNER.

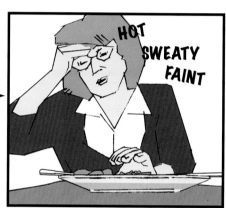

SINEMET PLUS

BREAKFAST
Porridge with fresh fruit

SINEMET PLUS & BETA BLOCKER

LUNCH
Soup with bread roll, and tomato salad

DINNER
Includes protein

SINEMET PLUS
Bed

I RAPIDLY FELT BETTER AND RETURNED THE DOSE TO A WHOLE TABLET THREE TIMES A DAY.

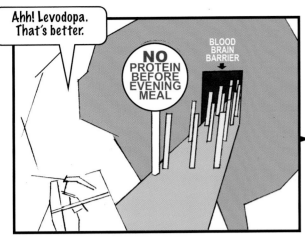

FOLLOWING A SHORT ROUTINE OF BURPS, SWEATS, SLEEP AND SNORTS I BEGAN A FOUR HOUR PERIOD OF FEELING **'UP'**
'UP' WAS WONDERFUL....

THE DRUGS BROUGHT BENEFITS TO MANY ASPECTS OF MY LIFE AND, IN THE CASE OF MUSCLE PAIN, REMOVED IT ALTOGETHER. HOWEVER, THE SIDE EFFECTS OF MY DRUGS STILL INCLUDED A DRY MOUTH, OCCASIONALLY A FASTER HEART RATE AND I DEVELOPED A RASH ON MY FOREHEAD THAT HAS NEVER GONE AWAY.

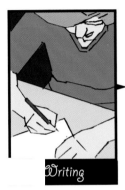
Writing

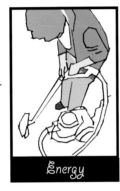
Energy

"Anyway, this was the first improvement since being diagnosed with Parkinson's more than five years earlier."

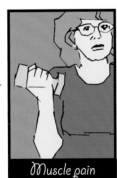
Stance

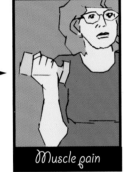
Muscle pain

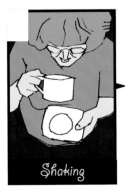
Shaking

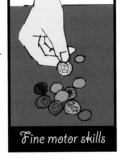
Fine motor skills

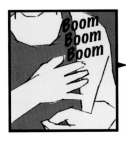

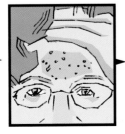

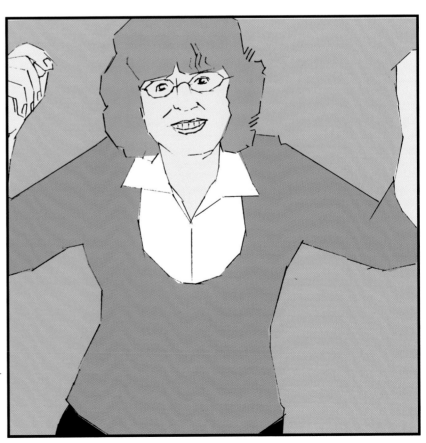

I HAVE ALWAYS THOUGHT IT VERY IMPORTANT TO MONITOR AND RECORD THE EFFECTS OF PARKINSON'S DRUGS ON MY BEHAVIOUR BECAUSE DOCTORS AND CONSULTANTS CANNOT ALWAYS PREDICT THE SIDE EFFECTS.

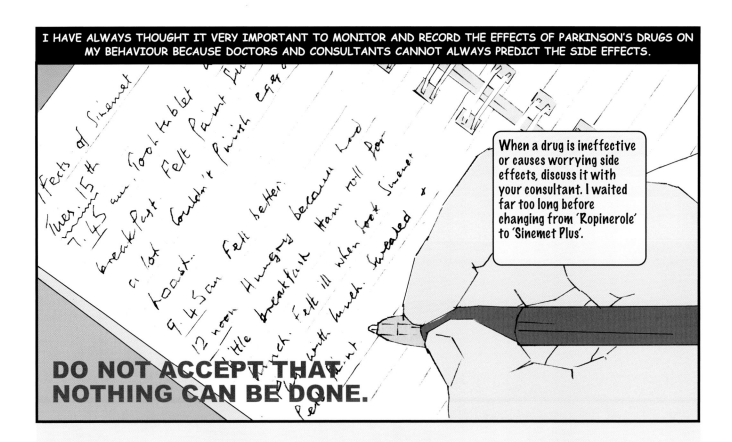

When a drug is ineffective or causes worrying side effects, discuss it with your consultant. I waited far too long before changing from 'Ropinerole' to 'Sinemet Plus'.

DO NOT ACCEPT THAT NOTHING CAN BE DONE.

It is equally important to take your drugs at the correct times.

During a stay in hospital I experience resistance from the hospital staff to me keeping my drugs.

IF YOU HAVE DIFFICULTIES, CONTACT YOUR CONSULTANT. IT WOULD ALSO BE WISE TO CONTACT PARKINSON'S UK FOR ADVICE BEFORE GOING INTO HOSPITAL.

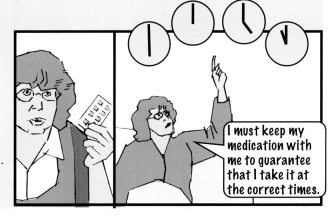

I must keep my medication with me to guarantee that I take it at the correct times.

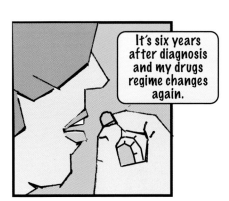

It's six years after diagnosis and my drugs regime changes again.

SO, I HAD BEEN TAKING SINEMET PLUS FOR ABOUT A YEAR AND THE **SIDE EFFECTS** (BURPS, SWEATS, SLEEP, SNORTS AND FASTER HEART RATE) HAD ALMOST DISAPPEARED. BUT THERE WAS A WORRYING INCREASE IN MY PARKINSON'S SYMPTOMS. I WAS WORKING PART-TIME.
MY CONSULTANT SUGGESTED I START TAKING FOUR TABLETS A DAY TO COUNTER THESE SYMPTOMS. THINGS IMPROVED. **HOWEVER, THE INCREASED MEDICATION DID NOT *COMPLETELY* REMOVE THE SYMPTOMS....**

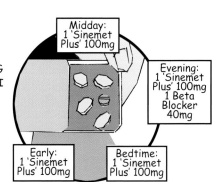

Midday:
1 'Sinemet
Plus' 100mg

Evening:
1 'Sinemet
Plus' 100mg
1 Beta
Blocker
40mg

Early:
1 'Sinemet
Plus' 100mg

Bedtime:
1 'Sinemet
Plus' 100mg

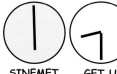
SINEMET PLUS
Taken in bed

GET UP

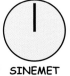
BREAKFAST
Porridge with fresh fruit

SINEMET PLUS

LUNCH
Soup with bread roll, and tomato salad

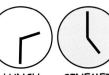
SINEMET PLUS & BETA BLOCKER

DINNER
Includes protein

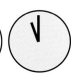
SINEMET PLUS
Bed

'UP' WAS BETTER AND I ENJOYED THE BENEFITS DESCRIBED EARLIER, BUT I STILL FELT THE EFFECTS OF PARKINSON'S, ESPECIALLY WHEN AT WORK. FOR EXAMPLE: CARRYING CASES, PUSHING OPEN DOORS, CLIMBING STAIRS AND THERE WAS ALWAYS SOME RESIDUAL SHAKING. **THE ONLY TIME SYMPTOMS COMPLETELY DISAPPEARED WAS WHEN THE MEDICATION WAS WORKING AND I WAS SITTING OR LYING DOWN.** OF COURSE, WHEN I WAS 'DOWN' OR GOING 'DOWN' OR IF THE MEDICATION FAILED TO WORK WHEN IT SHOULD, I FELT DISABLED. SO, I WAS IN A QUANDARY....

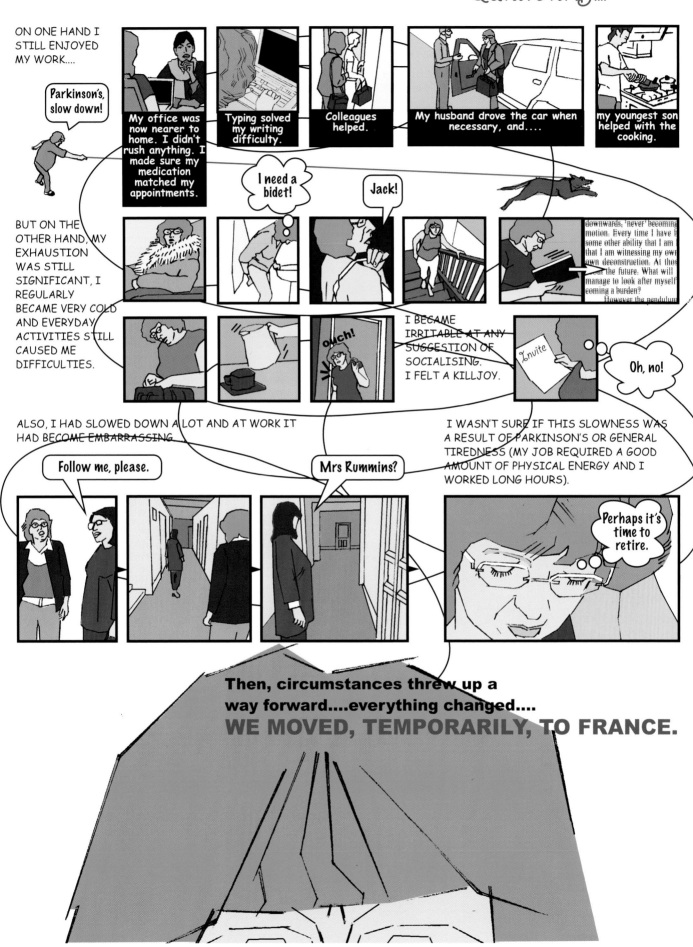

MY MOTHER WAS FRENCH AND I HAD BEEN TO SCHOOL IN PARIS FOR TWO YEARS AS A CHILD. IT WAS A COUNTRY WITH WHICH I HAD A STRONG CONNECTION AND BECAUSE OF THIS WE HAD ACQUIRED A SMALL HOUSE IN THE FRENCH COUNTRYSIDE. JUST THE PLACE TO GO, TO:

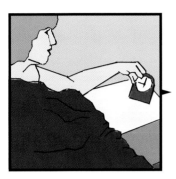

'LIE IN' AND DECIDE WHAT WAS TIREDNESS AND WHAT WAS PARKINSON'S.

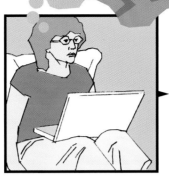

RELAX AND THINK OVER THE WORK SITUATION AND MAKE SOME PLANS FOR THE FUTURE....

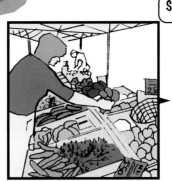

PRACTICE LIVING ON A REDUCED INCOME, AND....

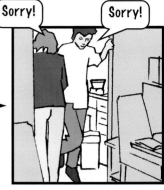

Sorry!

Sorry!

GIVE OUR YOUNGEST SON SOME SPACE FOR A YEAR, IN OUR SMALL LONDON FLAT, TO DO EXTRA STUDIES.

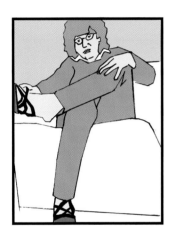

I wonder how Parkinson's will affect my French? I've already noticed that when I become tired, English words are hard to find and my train of thought is interrupted.

I 've also been referred to a speech therapist because my speech is too quiet.

So, how will the French respond to my shaking?

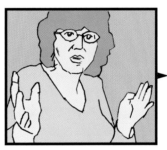

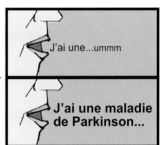

J'ai une...ummm

J'ai une maladie de Parkinson...

A N D   S O

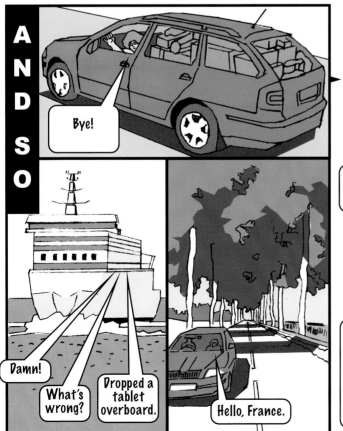

Bye!

Damn!

What's wrong?

Dropped a tablet overboard.

Hello, France.

OUR SMALL HOUSE IS ISOLATED ON THE EDGE OF A HAMLET, 5KM FROM THE NEAREST VILLAGE. **DURING OUR FIRST NIGHT.......**

PROWLERS!!!

Whats that noise?

Sounds like...

I'm calling the Police!

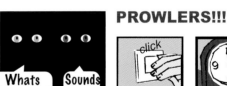

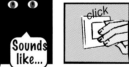

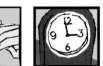

click

THREE GENDARMES SOON ARRIVED...

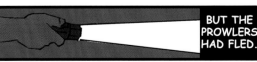

BUT THE PROWLERS HAD FLED.

You did the right thing madame.. *Thinks: Mon Dieu, she's nervous! Don't hesitate.. It's why we are here..*

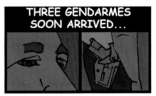

THE OFFICERS WERE EXTREMELY CONCERNED AND REASSURING. THEN I REALISED THAT I HAD NOT EXPLAINED MY SHAKING!

16

ONE OF THE MAJOR CHARACTERISTICS OF PARKINSON'S IS SLOWNESS OF MOVEMENT.

BEING IN FRANCE MEANT I HAD NO PRESSURE FROM WORK AND ALL THE TIME IN THE WORLD TO DO THINGS. IT SOON BECAME CLEAR THAT I HAD BECOME MUCH SLOWER THAN OTHER PEOPLE....

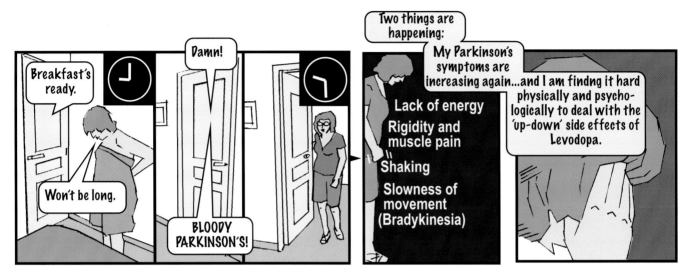

'UP-DOWN' IS HOW I EXPRESS FEELING 'UP' WHEN MY MEDICATION IS WORKING AND FEELING 'DOWN' WHEN IT WEARS OFF. WE RETURNED TO ENGLAND FOR CHRISTMAS AND IN JANUARY, SEVEN YEARS AFTER DIAGNOSIS AND TWO YEARS AFTER STARTING 'SINEMET PLUS' MY CONSULTANT INCREASED MY DOSE TO FIVE TABLETS A DAY.

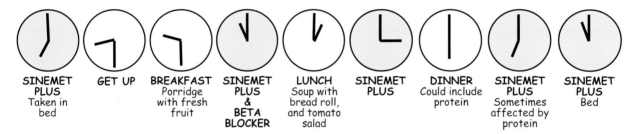

THIS MEANT THAT 'UP-DOWN' HAPPENED 5 TIMES A DAY. IT CONTROLLED MY LIFE.

When I am 'up', I get improvements in: Writing, Energy, Stance, Muscle pain, Shaking, Fine motor skills.

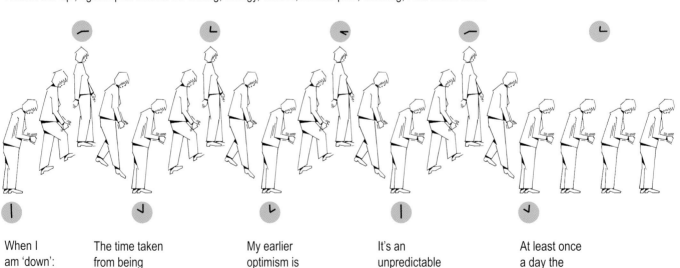

When I am 'down': The time taken from being 'halfway down' to 'down' can be as little as 20 minutes and in that time I feel I age 20 years. My earlier optimism is drowned in exhaustion. It's an unpredictable world with no sense of continuity, making it hard to plan anything. At least once a day the drugs don't work and I stay 'down'!

17

I HAD BEEN AWARE FOR A LONG TIME THAT PEOPLE FOUND IT DIFFICULT TO UNDERSTAND THAT I COULD DO SOMETHING ONE MINUTE, BUT NOT THE NEXT. IT WOULD HAVE BEEN NATURAL FOR PEOPLE TO THINK THAT I WAS EXAGGERATING. UNFORTUNATELY, SOME PEOPLE MADE REMARKS THAT WERE MEANT TO BE REASSURING BUT WHICH MADE ME ANGRY....

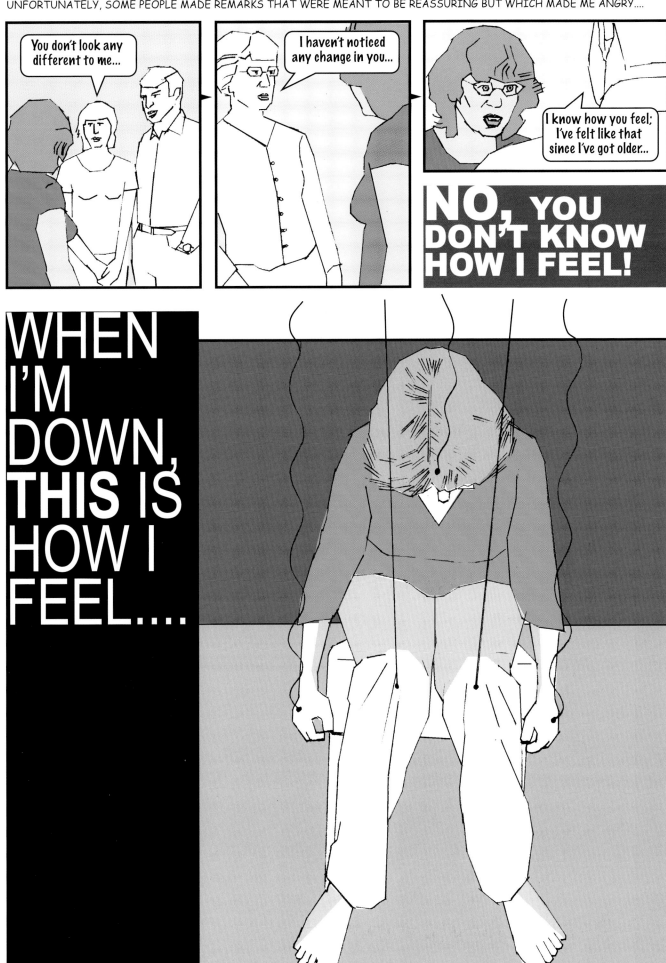

That Christmas, in England, turned out to be decision time....

IN FRANCE I HAD BEEN FINDING IT HARD TO PREDICT HOW WELL I WOULD FEEL FROM HOUR TO HOUR.

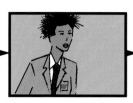

THIS WAS NOT COMPATIBLE WITH MY PROFESSIONAL RESPONSIBILITIES....

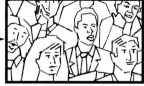

SO, I MADE THE DIFFICULT DECISION TO LOWER THE CURTAIN ON MY CAREER.

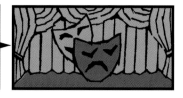

DURING THE CHRISTMAS HOLIDAY I WAS OFFERED NEW AND INTERESTING WORK.....

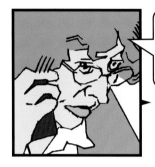

Sorry! I'm not taking on any new work because of my Parkinson's....

Yes, I've given it a lot of thought and that's my decision.

Thankyou-Goodbye!

SO, WHAT NEXT?

WRITING HAD ALWAYS BEEN AN INTEREST AND I HAD HALF WRITTEN A NOVEL (ABANDONED THROUGH LACK OF TIME).

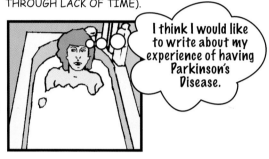

I think I would like to write about my experience of having Parkinson's Disease.

I WAS ALSO KEEN TO IMPROVE MY FRENCH BUT MORE IMPORTANTLY I SHOCKED EVERYONE BY DECLARING....

I'm going to do something I've always wanted to do- learn to cook properly...

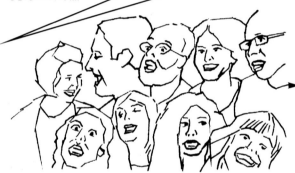

UP TO THIS POINT I HAD WORKED, RETURNED TO STUDIES, EMBARKED ON A NEW CAREER AND RAISED A FAMILY. THIS DID NOT LEAVE TIME FOR FANCY COOKING. (LUCKILY, MY SONS BECAME VERY GOOD COOKS AT A YOUNG AGE).

I AM NATURALLY A SOCIABLE PERSON WHO ENJOYS COMMUNICATING. SO, ENTERTAINING PEOPLE AT HOME WITHOUT RESORTING TO SUPERMARKET 'READYMEALS' WAS OF BENEFIT TO EVERYONE. IT ALSO SAVED ME THE AWKWARDNESS AND EMBARRASSMENT THAT ACCOMPANIED EAING OUT....

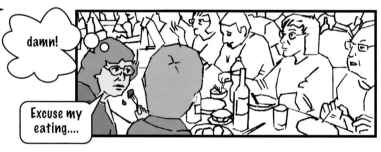

damn!

Excuse my eating....

SO FAR, SO GOOD.

BUT THE FINE MOTOR SKILLS THAT WERE REQUIRED TO PEEL, CHOP AND CUT WERE A PROBLEM. I HAD FOUND OTHER WAYS OF DOING THESE JOBS, BUT I STILL LACKED SUFFICIENT GRIP TO USE SOME UTENSILS EVEN WHEN FEELING 'UP'. NEVERTHELESS, I REARRANGED THE KITCHEN (WITH HELP) AND BOUGHT A SIMPLE FOOD MIXER FOR BEATING AND MIXING.

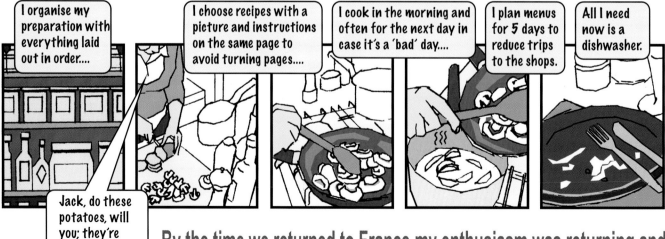

I organise my preparation with everything laid out in order....

I choose recipes with a picture and instructions on the same page to avoid turning pages....

I cook in the morning and often for the next day in case it's a 'bad' day....

I plan menus for 5 days to reduce trips to the shops.

All I need now is a dishwasher.

Jack, do these potatoes, will you; they're exhausting me...

By the time we returned to France my enthusiasm was returning and I was daring to think that my future might possibly look meaningful.

But what about these problems with movement?
Parkinson's can be described medically as a movement disorder.

I HAD MORE PROBLEMS WITH MY FINE MOTOR SKILLS (SMALL, FIDDLY MOVEMENTS) THAN I DID WITH MY GROSS MOTOR SKILLS (LARGE MOVEMENTS LIKE WALKING).

MY SPATIAL PERCEPTION WAS POOR WHICH AFFECTED MY BALANCE AND SO I HAD TO BE CAREFUL TO DO THINGS AT MY PACE.

FORTUNATELY, I DIDN'T SUFFER FROM 'FREEZING' WHEN ATTEMPTING TO WALK OR HAVE A DIFFICULTY IN STOPPING ONCE I HAD STARTED - LIKE MANY SUFFERERS.

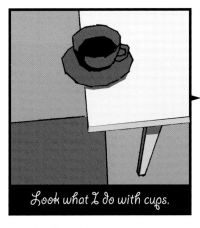

Look what I do with cups.

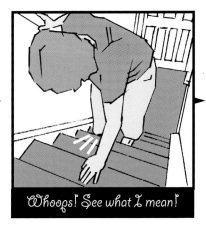

Whoops! See what I mean!

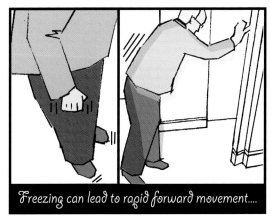

Freezing can lead to rapid forward movement....

Initiating some movements, however, were a problem for me...

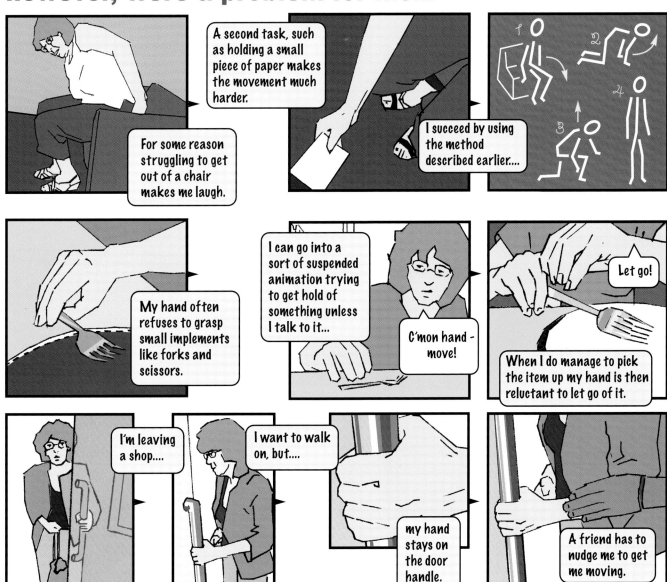

For some reason struggling to get out of a chair makes me laugh.

A second task, such as holding a small piece of paper makes the movement much harder.

I succeed by using the method described earlier....

My hand often refuses to grasp small implements like forks and scissors.

I can go into a sort of suspended animation trying to get hold of something unless I talk to it...

C'mon hand - move!

Let go!

When I do manage to pick the item up my hand is then reluctant to let go of it.

I'm leaving a shop....

I want to walk on, but....

my hand stays on the door handle.

A friend has to nudge me to get me moving.

20

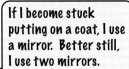

If I become stuck putting on a coat, I use a mirror. Better still, I use two mirrors.

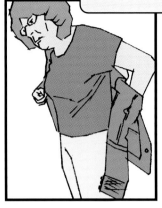

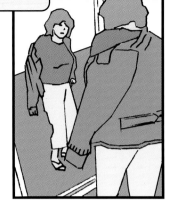

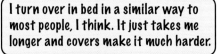

I turn over in bed in a similar way to most people, I think. It just takes me longer and covers make it much harder.

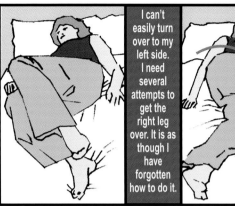

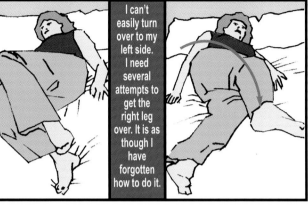

I can't easily turn over to my left side. I need several attempts to get the right leg over. It is as though I have forgotten how to do it.

Fine motor movements were steadily becoming more difficult to carry out.

THE FOLLOWING SITUATION ILLUSTRATES THIS PROBLEM:

My right arm and hand often feel like a......

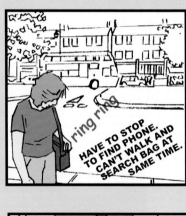

ring ring — HAVE TO STOP TO FIND PHONE. CAN'T WALK AND SEARCH BAG AT SAME TIME.

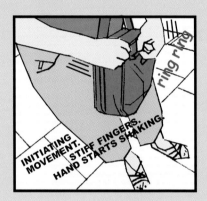

ring ring — INITIATING MOVEMENT. STIFF FINGERS. HAND STARTS SHAKING.

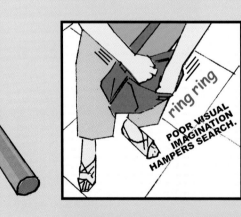

ring ring — POOR VISUAL IMAGINATION HAMPERS SEARCH.

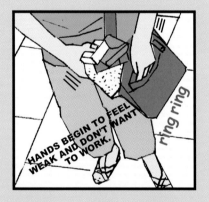

ring ring — HANDS BEGIN TO FEEL WEAK AND DON'T WANT TO WORK.

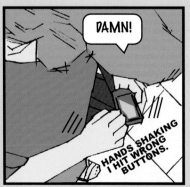

DAMN! — HANDS SHAKING I HIT WRONG BUTTONS.

IN THIS SITUATION I SELDOM REACH THE PHONE IN TIME TO ANSWER IT.

My solution to fine motor difficulties:
1. Break the task into small parts.
2. Practice each part.
3. Only attempt one action at a time.
4. Try to keep relaxed.
5. If unsuccessful - rest and try again later.

21

WHEN I FIRST DEVELOPED PARKINSON'S, BEFORE IT HAD BEEN DIAGNOSED, I THOUGHT MY SYMPTOMS WERE AS THE RESULT OF STRESS. SO....

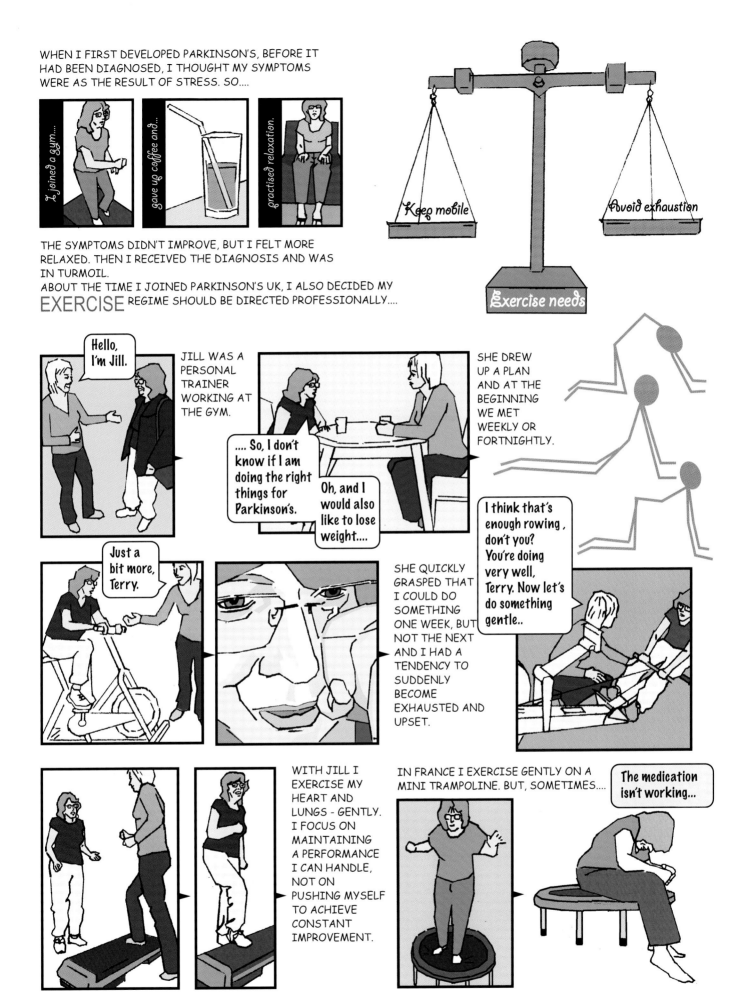

I joined a gym....

gave up coffee and...

practised relaxation.

Keep mobile — **Avoid exhaustion**

Exercise needs

THE SYMPTOMS DIDN'T IMPROVE, BUT I FELT MORE RELAXED. THEN I RECEIVED THE DIAGNOSIS AND WAS IN TURMOIL.
ABOUT THE TIME I JOINED PARKINSON'S UK, I ALSO DECIDED MY EXERCISE REGIME SHOULD BE DIRECTED PROFESSIONALLY....

Hello, I'm Jill.

JILL WAS A PERSONAL TRAINER WORKING AT THE GYM.

.... So, I don't know if I am doing the right things for Parkinson's.

Oh, and I would also like to lose weight....

SHE DREW UP A PLAN AND AT THE BEGINNING WE MET WEEKLY OR FORTNIGHTLY.

Just a bit more, Terry.

SHE QUICKLY GRASPED THAT I COULD DO SOMETHING ONE WEEK, BUT NOT THE NEXT AND I HAD A TENDENCY TO SUDDENLY BECOME EXHAUSTED AND UPSET.

I think that's enough rowing, don't you? You're doing very well, Terry. Now let's do something gentle..

WITH JILL I EXERCISE MY HEART AND LUNGS - GENTLY. I FOCUS ON MAINTAINING A PERFORMANCE I CAN HANDLE, NOT ON PUSHING MYSELF TO ACHIEVE CONSTANT IMPROVEMENT.

IN FRANCE I EXERCISE GENTLY ON A MINI TRAMPOLINE. BUT, SOMETIMES....

The medication isn't working...

CARDIOVASCULAR EXERCISE IS VERY IMPORTANT NOW THAT I HAVE SLOWED DOWN SO MUCH AND GET LESS EXERCISE FROM NORMAL DAILY ACTIVITIES SUCH AS WALKING.

I ALSO WORKED ON MY POSTURE AND BALANCE TO MAKE ME MORE STEADY ON MY FEET AND GIVE ME MORE CONFIDENCE IN MY MOVEMENTS....

SOMETIMES THIS WAS AS SIMPLE AS GOING FOR A WALK WITH JILL, BUT USUALLY I FOLLOWED ONE OF THE GENTLE EXERCISES SHE HAD DESIGNED FOR ME. THESE EXERCISES WERE OFTEN DONE WHILST LOOKING IN A MIRROR WHICH HELPED MY SPATIAL AWARENESS AND THEREFORE MY MOVEMENT CONTROL.

Jill and I became good friends. Professionally, she was all a good personal trainer should be: patient, encouraging and focused on her client. She has done wonders for my self-esteem. Our relationship has now lasted several years.

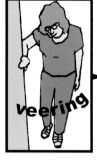

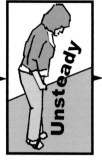

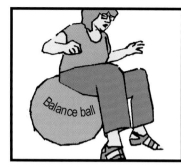

Shall we go a little faster...

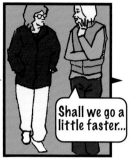

Balance ball

A FURTHER AREA OF EXERCISE IS STRETCHING. THIS HELPS PREVENT PAINFUL STIFFNESS IN MY RIGHT ARM FROM THE SHOULDER TO THE WRIST THAT CAUSES MY HAND TO CLENCH. ONCE OR TWICE A DAY JACK PULLS MY ARM FOR ABOUT 20 SECONDS, DOING THIS 2 OR 3 TIMES. THIS STRETCHING CAN PREVENT STIFFNESS HAPPENING OR, IF I AM SUFFERING PAIN, IT CAN ALLEVIATE IT.

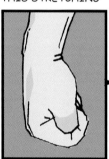

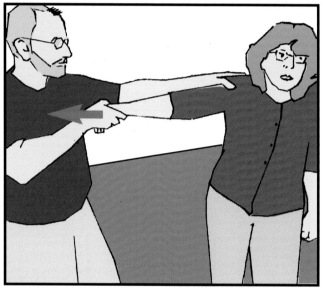

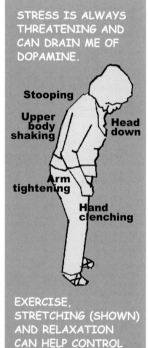

STRESS IS ALWAYS THREATENING AND CAN DRAIN ME OF DOPAMINE.

Stooping

Upper body shaking

Head down

Arm tightening

Hand clenching

LARGE MOVEMENTS ARE EASIER THAN SMALL ONES.

SO, FOR EXAMPLE, WHEN I FIND IT HARD TO INITIATE MOVEMENT, SAY TO GET OUT OF A CHAIR OR TO START WRITING (BECAUSE MY RIGHT ARM MUSCLES ARE TIGHT), I SURPRISE MYSELF BY BEING ABLE TO DRAW USING BIGGER MOVEMENTS.
I AM NOT AN ARTIST, BUT JACK, WHO IS AN ILLUSTRATOR, SUGGESTED SOME DRAWING EXERCISES THAT FORCED ME TO USE BIG MOVEMENTS TO FILL LARGE SHEETS OF PAPER.

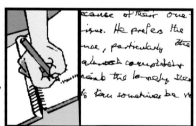

EXERCISE, STRETCHING (SHOWN) AND RELAXATION CAN HELP CONTROL STRESS.

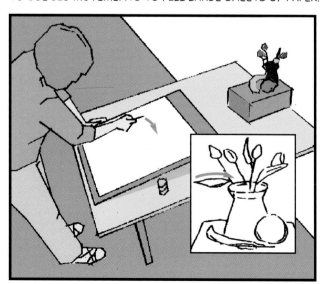

ALTHOUGH I HAVE DECREASED MY EXERCISE BECAUSE OF THE TIREDNESS FACTOR I STILL FOLLOW THE RULE THAT SAYS....

TO KEEP MOBILE YOU HAVE TO KEEP MOVING.

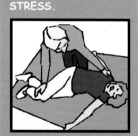

IN FRANCE I JOINED A RELAXATION CLASS ARRANGED BY THE LOCAL PARKINSON'S GROUP. I FOUND THIS HELPED MY GENERAL WELL-BEING.

I HAVE HAD MAINLY POSITIVE EXPERIENCES OF SLEEPING DURING THE TIME I HAVE HAD PARKINSON'S....

BEFORE DIAGNOSIS.

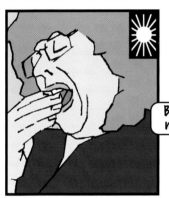

Light sleep, sometimes disturbed with waking dreams.

DIAGNOSIS OF PARKINSON'S.

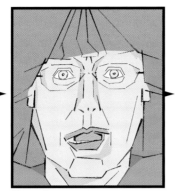

Turmoil.

6 MONTHS AFTER DIAGNOSIS.

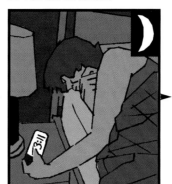

Bad sleep, but waking dreams became less frequent, and then ceased. *Medication: Agonist.*

6 MONTHS - 18 MONTHS

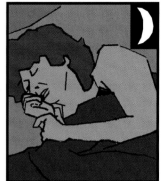

Normal to very good sleep. *Medication: Agonist+ Amytriptyline.*

18 MONTHS TO PRESENT.

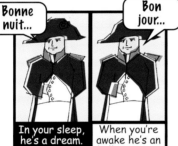

Normal/heavy to very good sleep with some disruptive daytime sleepiness. *Medication: Agonist replaced by Levodopa.*

I WAS WARNED, AS I EMBARKED ON LEVODOPA, THAT I MAY GET HALLUCINATIONS. LUCKILY, I NEVER DID BUT WHAT DID CHANGE WAS THAT I BEGAN REMEMBERING MY DREAMS FAR MORE OFTEN.

Bonne nuit...

Bon jour...

In your sleep, he's a dream.

When you're awake he's an hallucination.

IN FRANCE, RECENT PARKINSON'S LITERATURE HAS FOCUSED ON SCREENING TO FOREWARN OF THE DEVELOPMENT OF THE DISEASE. SOME CHARACTERISTICS HAVE BEEN IDENTIFIED THAT MIGHT BE IMPORTANT IN THIS RESPECT....

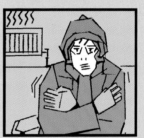

Fluctuations in body temperature. *I experienced this.*

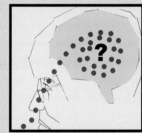

Loss of sense of smell. *I didn't experience this but now, I sometimes smell things that aren't there like smokey fires on television.*

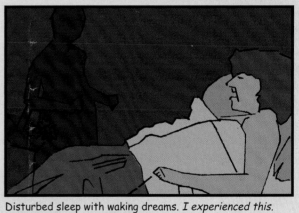

Disturbed sleep with waking dreams. *I experienced this.*

TWO FACTORS WHICH CONTRIBUTE TO MY DISTURBED SLEEP ARE:

1 Shaking

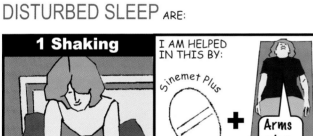

I AM HELPED IN THIS BY:

Sinemet Plus + *Arms relax...*

2 Stiffness

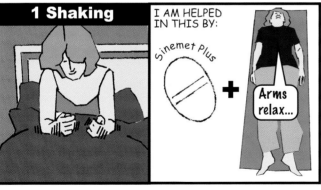

I AM HELPED IN THIS BY:

Sinemet Plus + *Legs relax...* +

How's that?

...and also by having my arm shaken randomly.

Lovely - will you pull it again.

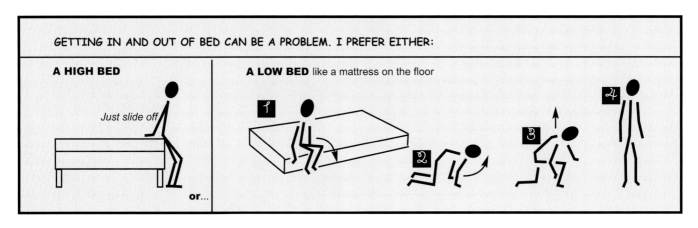

GETTING IN AND OUT OF BED CAN BE A PROBLEM. I PREFER EITHER:

A HIGH BED

Just slide off

A LOW BED like a mattress on the floor

or...

EXHAUSTION IS ANOTHER EVER-PRESENT THEME.
AN ACQUAINTANCE IN MY LOCAL FRENCH PARKINSON'S GROUP TOLD ME THAT THE MORE SHE SLEEPS THE LESS HER PARKINSON'S SYMPTOMS TROUBLE HER WHEN SHE IS AWAKE.
I MAKE SURE I HAVE ENOUGH SATISFYING SLEEP....

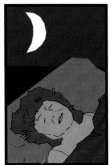 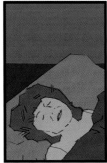 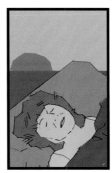 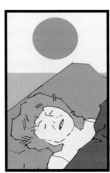 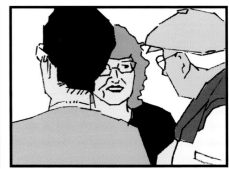

THEN I CAN STILL ENJOY LIFE.

ON THE FEW OCCASIONS I HAVE BECOME DEPRESSED IT WAS BECAUSE I WAS OVER-TIRED, COLD AND HUNGRY.
THIS WAS MY REMEDY:

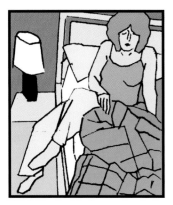 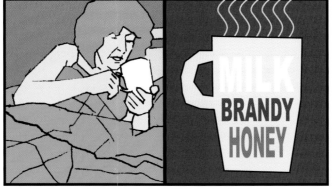 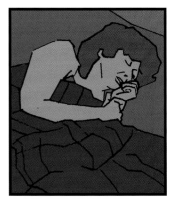

MILK
BRANDY
HONEY

I DON'T SHAKE
WHEN ASLEEP.
IF I DAYDREAM I
DON'T SHAKE
EITHER.

FOR EXAMPLE, IF I DAYDREAM
ABOUT THE AREA OF FRANCE
WE GO TO, I DON'T SHAKE.
UNFORTUNATELY, AS SOON
AS I BECOME AWARE THAT I
AM DAYDREAMING, I START
SHAKING AGAIN.

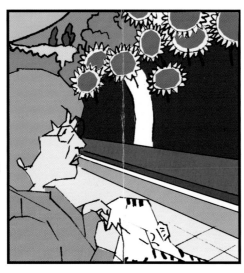

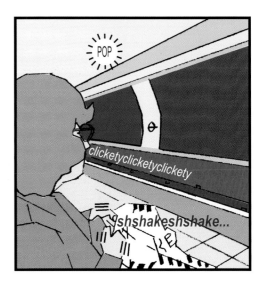

POP

clicketyclicketyclickety

shshakeshshake...

25

I'VE ALWAYS ENJOYED COMMUNICATING

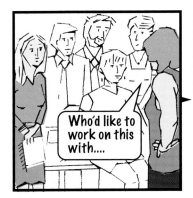

"Who'd like to work on this with...."

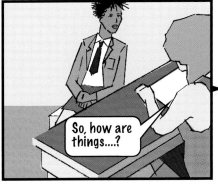

"So, how are things....?"

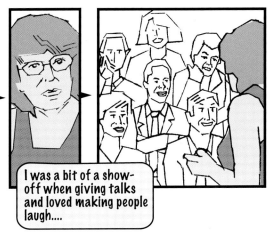

"I was a bit of a show-off when giving talks and loved making people laugh...."

SO, IT WAS WORRYING WHEN NEARLY SEVEN YEARS AFTER DIAGNOSIS, MY SPEECH BECAME HALTING AND UNSURE. BECAUSE OF MY SHAKING I THOUGHT I WAS BECOMING SELF-CONSCIOUS. BUT, IT GOT WORSE.....

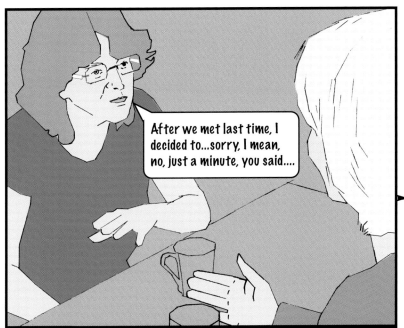

"After we met last time, I decided to...sorry, I mean, no, just a minute, you said...."

My speech was too quiet and my words would tumble over each other. I lost sensitivity and humour. Sometimes I had difficulty in finding words. I was losing the ability to emit and pronounce words in an acceptable time period.

THIS INDISTINCTNESS SEEMED TO BE A PRONUNCIATION PROBLEM AND AS SUCH I THOUGHT IT MUST BE A MOTOR DIFFICULTY.

GOING TO FRANCE AND SPEAKING FRENCH HAS FORCED ME TO CONCENTRATE ON PRONUNCIATION AND DICTION. I HAVE ALSO EXPANDED MY VOCABULARY (SO, NO PROBLEM WITH MY MEMORY).

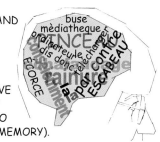

THIS ATTENTION TO ANOTHER LANGUAGE HAS GIVEN ME MORE CONFIDENCE WHEN SPEAKING ENGLISH. I'M CAREFUL TO KEEP....

MY VOICE....	MY SPEECH....	MY WORDS....
LOUD ENOUGH	SLO WW WW ENO..	kleer i-nuf

ANOTHER ASPECT OF COMMUNICATION IS FACIAL EXPRESSION. I HAVE SOME LACK OF FLEXIBILITY ON THE RIGHT SIDE OF MY FACE. SO, I NOW PRACTISE FACE MUSCLE EXERCISES. HERE ARE SOME EXAMPLES....

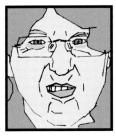
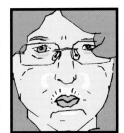
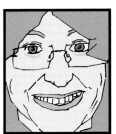
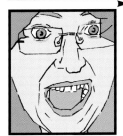

FOR ME, COMMUNICATION KEEPS FRIENDSHIPS ALIVE, STARTS NEW FRIENDSHIPS AND PRESERVES A SENSE OF PERSPECTIVE.
LACK OF COMMUNICATION ENCOURAGES ME TO WITHDRAW AND BE SAD.

PROBABLY THE MOST IMPORTANT FACTOR ABOUT COMMUNICATION WITH OTHER PEOPLE IS TO *KEEP DOING IT -* WHATEVER THE DIFFICULTY.....

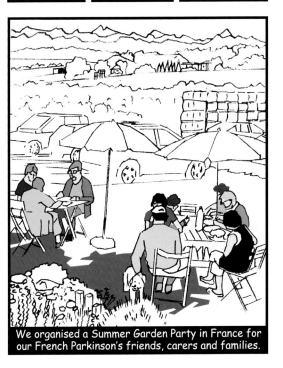

We organised a Summer Garden Party in France for our French Parkinson's friends, carers and families.

MY ORIGINAL AIM IN WRITING THIS STORY WAS TO GIVE PEOPLE WHO HAD RECEIVED A DIAGNOSIS OF PARKINSON'S SOME IDEA OF HOW THE DISEASE HAD AFFECTED ANOTHER PERSON; ME.

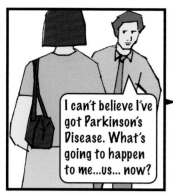

I NOW REALISE THAT I HAVE ALSO BEEN WRITING FOR MANY OTHERS, INCLUDING MYSELF....

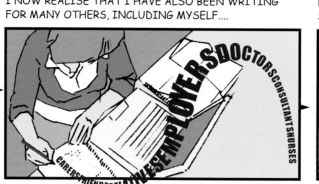

I can't believe I've got Parkinson's Disease. What's going to happen to me...us... now?

FIRSTLY, I WAS SHOCKED AND SURPRISED BY MY DIAGNOSIS.

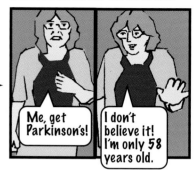

Me, get Parkinson's!

I don't believe it! I'm only 58 years old.

THEN MY **FEELINGS** MOVED TO ANGER, UPSET, SELF-PITY, ENVY, JEALOUSY AND HOPELESSNESS ABOUT THE FUTURE, **BUT**....

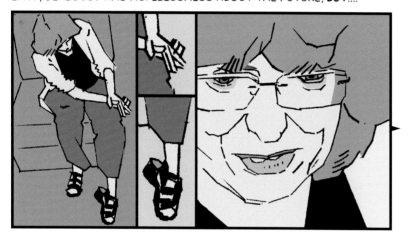

I ALSO FELT GRATITUDE TO THE MEDICAL PROFESSION....

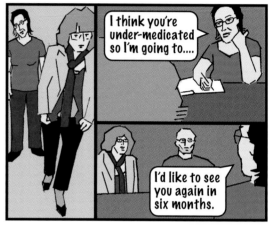

I think you're under-medicated so I'm going to....

I'd like to see you again in six months.

I FELT SUPPORTED AND BECAME USED TO HAVING PARKINSON'S. BUT, ABOUT SEVEN YEARS AFTER DIAGNOSIS, EXHAUSTION KICKED IN AND MY MOTOR SKILLS WORSENED SIGNIFICANTLY. I DISCOVERED THAT PARKINSON'S MEANT BUSINESS...

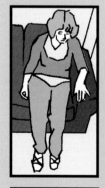

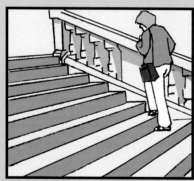

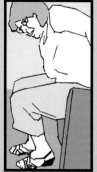

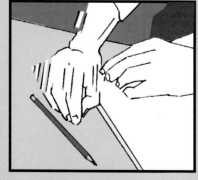

THIS WAS THE DETERIORATING CONDITION I HAD BEEN TOLD ABOUT. I REALISED, FOR EXAMPLE, THAT I MAY *NEVER* BE ABLE TO HANDWRITE A PAGE OF NOTES AGAIN.

NEVER WAS A SCARY WORD TO USE. I ASSOCIATED IT WITH GIVING UP; A CUL DE SAC; A DEAD END....

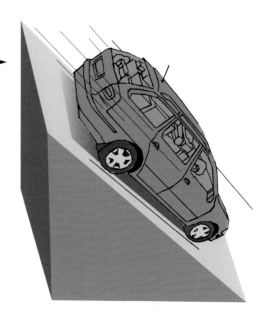

THERE WAS A DANGER, AS PARKINSON'S DEVELOPED, FOR ME TO BECOME RIGID, BOTH PHYSICALLY AND EMOTIONALLY, BY HOLDING ON TO THINGS I COULD CONTROL. AS I LOST ABILITIES I WORRIED ABOUT THE FUTURE. WHAT WOULD HAPPEN TO ME? ONE OFTEN HEARS THAT ONE MUST LEARN TO **ACCEPT** PARKINSON'S, BUT I PREFERRED THE CONCEPT OF TRANSFORMATION~ TURNING A NEGATIVE SITUATION INTO A POSITIVE ONE.

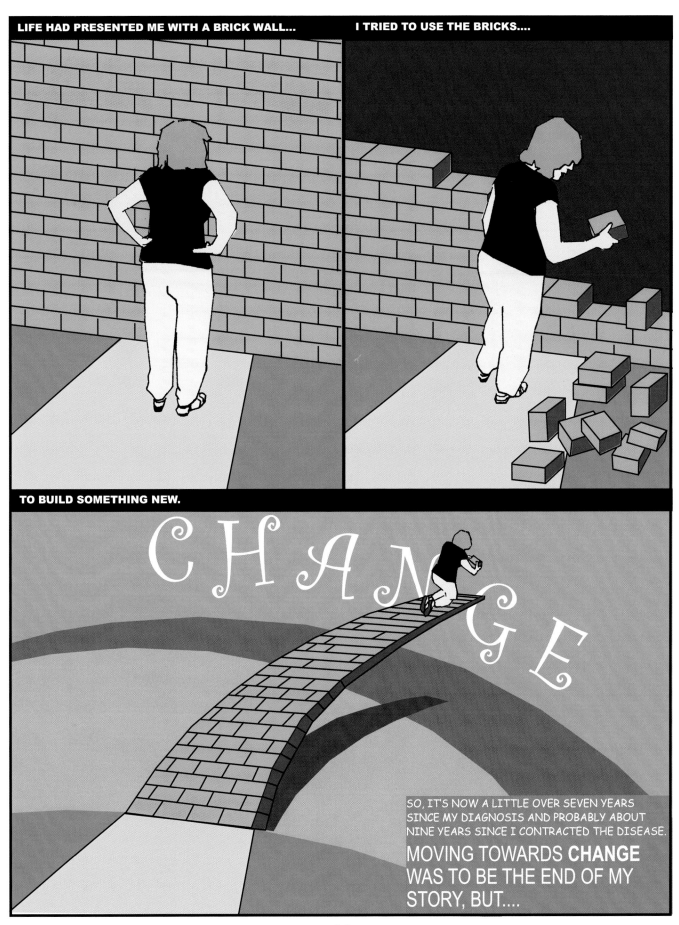

LIFE HAD PRESENTED ME WITH A BRICK WALL...

I TRIED TO USE THE BRICKS....

TO BUILD SOMETHING NEW.

CHANGE

SO, IT'S NOW A LITTLE OVER SEVEN YEARS SINCE MY DIAGNOSIS AND PROBABLY ABOUT NINE YEARS SINCE I CONTRACTED THE DISEASE. MOVING TOWARDS **CHANGE** WAS TO BE THE END OF MY STORY, BUT....

Two years later....

The past two years have been a happy time. Almost by default I have accepted that I have Parkinson's. I didn't try to do so; my feelings just changed.

FOR A LONG TIME I HAVE USED AN APPROACH WHICH I HAVE FOUND VERY HELPFUL WHEN I HAVE A PROBLEM TO FACE AND WHEN ALL IDEAS I CAN THINK OF, FAIL TO SOLVE IT. THE APPROACH ASSUMES THAT DOING SOMETHING ABOUT A DIFFICULT SITUATION IS NOT NECESSARILY BETTER THAN DOING NOTHING ABOUT IT.

I HAD A DREAM THAT SUMMARISED THIS FOR ME....

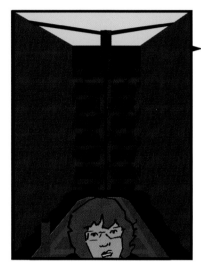

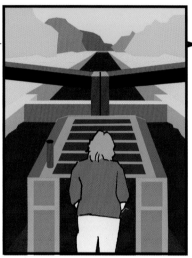

THIS APPROACH HAS DEVELOPED INTO WHAT I CALL 'CREATIVE INACTIVITY'.....

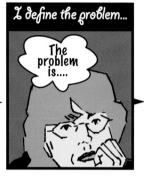

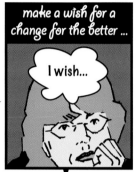

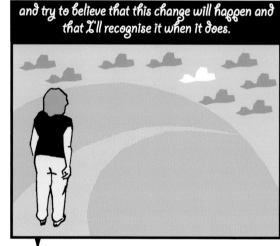

I WAS AT THE BOTTOM OF A DARK LOCK, IN A SMALL BOAT. I WAS FEELING DEPRESSED. SUDDENLY, I REALISED THAT IF I DID NOTHING AND GAVE THE SMALL BOAT TIME, THINGS WOULD CHANGE...

THE WATER IN THE LOCK ROSE AND THE BOAT EVENTUALLY REACHED THE TOP OF THE LOCK. I WAS NO LONGER DEPRESSED.

CHANGES IN LIFESTYLE AND MAKING NEW RELATIONSHIPS WERE MY ANTIDOTES TO RIGIDITY AND NEGATIVITY.

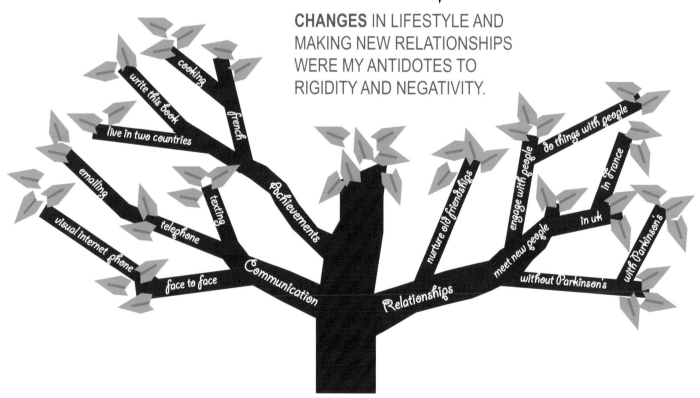

GIVING UP WORK BECAUSE OF PARKINSON'S WAS VERY HARD FOR ME, BUT EVENTUALLY I APPRECIATED THE EXTRA TIME I HAD. THIS LET ME.......

explore life in France and develop my french...

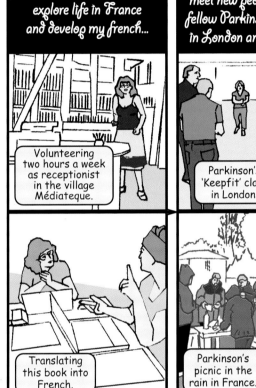

Volunteering two hours a week as receptionist in the village Médiateque.

Translating this book into French.

meet new people especially fellow Parkinson's sufferers in London and in France...

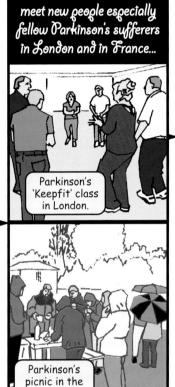

Parkinson's 'Keepfit' class in London.

Parkinson's picnic in the rain in France.

nurture old friendships and be with my family, especially my husband Jack...

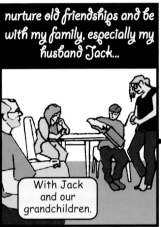

With Jack and our grandchildren.

improve my cooking.

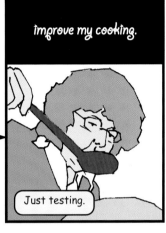

Just testing.

IN LONDON WE JOINED OUR LOCAL PARKINSON'S GROUP. WHICH RUNS MANY ACTIVITIES FROM KEEPFIT TO THEATRE VISITS. WE HAVE MADE MANY NEW FRIENDS.

Wii practise.

Alexander Technique session.

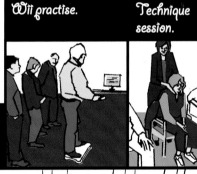

Drawing at one of our regular group meetings.

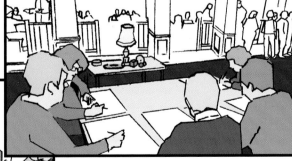

WE ALSO ATTEND A SEPARATE SINGING GROUP FOR PARKINSON'S SUFFERERS. I SHOULD SAY IMMEDIATELY THAT MINE IS NOT A SINGING VOICE BUT I LET RIP IN THE KNOWLEDGE THAT IT'S GOOD THERAPY FOR MY PARKINSON'S. OH, AND IT'S GREAT FUN.

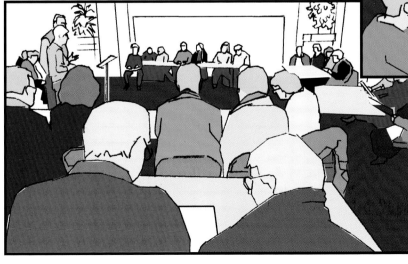

CHANGES IN MY LIFESTYLE HAVE ENSURED THAT I CAN CONTINUE HAVING PLANS AND PROJECTS AND LEAD A MEANINGFUL LIFE.

SO, HAVING PARKINSON'S DOES NOT INEVITABLY STOP ONE FROM BEING ONESELF AND ENJOYING ONESELF.

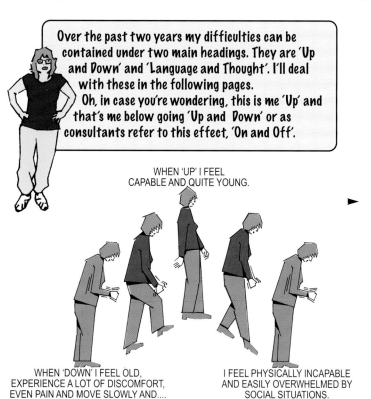

Over the past two years my difficulties can be contained under two main headings. They are 'Up and Down' and 'Language and Thought'. I'll deal with these in the following pages.
Oh, in case you're wondering, this is me 'Up' and that's me below going 'Up and Down' or as consultants refer to this effect, 'On and Off'.

WHEN 'UP' I FEEL CAPABLE AND QUITE YOUNG.

WHEN 'DOWN' I FEEL OLD, EXPERIENCE A LOT OF DISCOMFORT, EVEN PAIN AND MOVE SLOWLY AND....

I FEEL PHYSICALLY INCAPABLE AND EASILY OVERWHELMED BY SOCIAL SITUATIONS.

UP and DOWN is brought about by Parkinson's medication. Without Sinemet Plus I would always be 'down'. As time has gone by, I have found that the Up and Down effect has become more intense. My 'Ups' are now more dramatic and my 'Downs' are more extreme.
At present my medication takes me 'Up' six times a day and I come 'Down' six times a day....

MY MEDICATION IS....

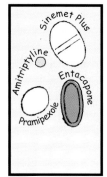

Sinemet Plus which includes Levodopa (this converts into Dopamine in the body).
Pramipexole a Dopamine Agonist that imitates the effects of Dopamine. It gives me a feeling of greater well-being.
Entacapone that slows the breakdown of Levodopa in the body making my 'Up' about 30 minutes longer.
Amitriptyline in small doses that helps me sleep.

EACH DAY I TAKE...

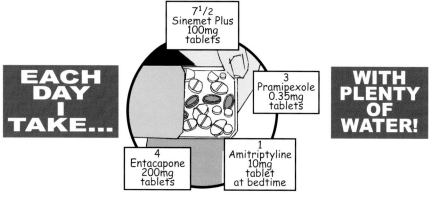

7 1/2 Sinemet Plus 100mg tablets

3 Pramipexole 0.35mg tablets

4 Entacapone 200mg tablets

1 Amitriptyline 10mg tablet at bedtime

WITH PLENTY OF WATER!

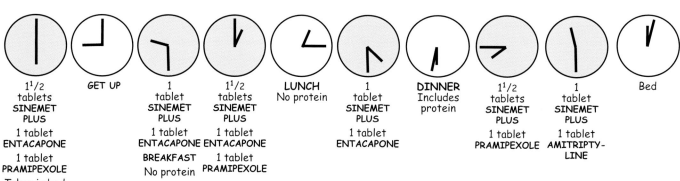

| 1 1/2 tablets SINEMET PLUS 1 tablet ENTACAPONE 1 tablet PRAMIPEXOLE Taken in bed | GET UP | 1 tablet SINEMET PLUS 1 tablet ENTACAPONE BREAKFAST No protein | 1 1/2 tablets SINEMET PLUS 1 tablet ENTACAPONE 1 tablet PRAMIPEXOLE | LUNCH No protein | 1 tablet SINEMET PLUS 1 tablet ENTACAPONE | DINNER Includes protein | 1 1/2 tablets SINEMET PLUS 1 tablet PRAMIPEXOLE | 1 tablet SINEMET PLUS 1 tablet AMITRIPTY-LINE | Bed |

SO, I GO 'UP' SIX TIMES A DAY AND I COME DOWN SIX TIMES A DAY.

WHEN EACH DOSE OF MEDICATION STARTS WORKING, I GO 'UP' AND AS EACH DOSE STOPS WORKING I COME 'DOWN'. SOMETIMES A DOSE DOES NOT WORK AT ALL AND I STAY DOWN.

ALL OF WHICH MEANS....

I MOVE FROM ONE PERSONALITY TO ANOTHER PERSONALITY SEVERAL TIMES A DAY. I HAVE TO ADJUST TO THESE CHANGES. IN THE NORMAL COURSE OF EVENTS THIS DOESN'T DEPRESS ME BECAUSE WHEN I'M 'DOWN' I KNOW THAT IN MOST CASES I WILL COME 'UP' AGAIN. EQUALLY, WHEN 'UP' I HAVE LEARNED NOT TO COMMIT MYSELF TO TASKS I PROBABLY CANNOT FULFIL BECAUSE I KNOW I WILL GO 'DOWN' AGAIN. NOWADAYS, I SOMETIMES GO EXTREMELY 'DOWN'. IN THIS SITUATION I USE MY SECRET WEAPON - AT LEAST 30 MINUTES OF TOTAL REST.
UNFORTUNATELY, I AM NOT ALWAYS SOMEWHERE WHERE THIS IS POSSIBLE.....

UP

Writing a shopping list....

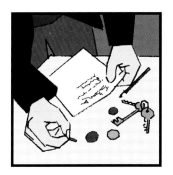

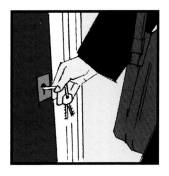

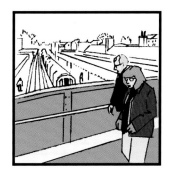

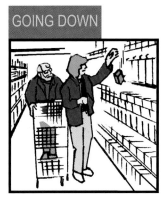

GOING DOWN

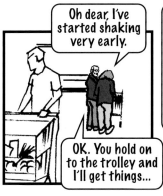

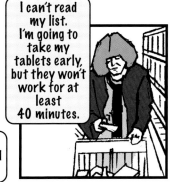

Oh dear, I've started shaking very early.

OK. You hold on to the trolley and I'll get things...

I can't read my list. I'm going to take my tablets early, but they won't work for at least 40 minutes.

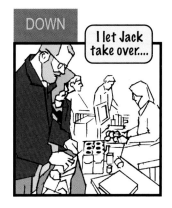

DOWN

I let Jack take over....

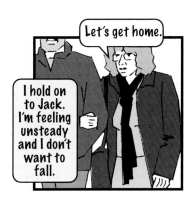

Let's get home.

I hold on to Jack. I'm feeling unsteady and I don't want to fall.

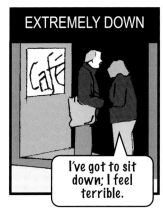

EXTREMELY DOWN

I've got to sit down; I feel terrible.

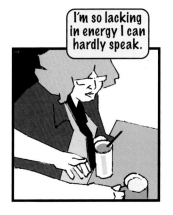

I'm so lacking in energy I can hardly speak.

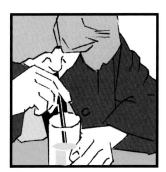

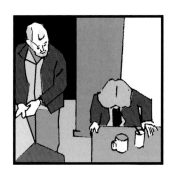

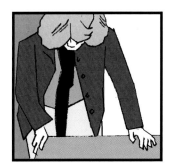

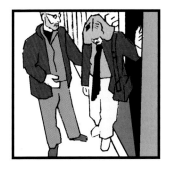

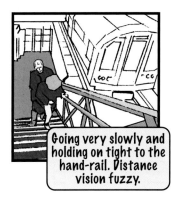

Going very slowly and holding on tight to the hand-rail. Distance vision fuzzy.

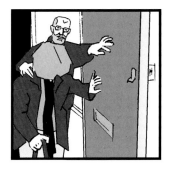

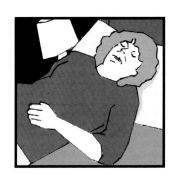

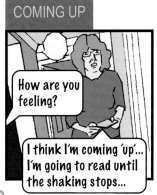

COMING UP

How are you feeling?

I think I'm coming 'up'... I'm going to read until the shaking stops...

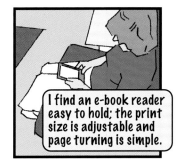

I find an e-book reader easy to hold; the print size is adjustable and page turning is simple.

TWO YEARS AGO I MENTIONED SOME LACK OF FLEXIBILITY IN MY FACE.

THIS HAS INCREASED SLIGHTLY, BUT I CAN STILL SHOW MY FEELINGS, SUCH AS SYMPATHY, JOY AND EXCITEMENT USING FACIAL EXPRESSION ~ MANY CAN'T.

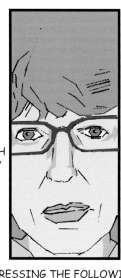

HOWEVER, MY SPEECH HAS DETERIORATED MORE. THE AMOUNT OF DETERIORATION DEPENDS ON WHETHER I AM 'UP' OR 'DOWN'. IF 'DOWN' I AVOID LONG, DETAILED OR STRESSFUL CONVERSATIONS. IF I DON'T THE EFFORT PRODUCES NOT ONLY SHAKING, BUT....

A weak voice...

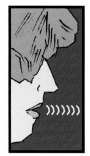

A difficulty in pronouncing varied 'syllable sounds' such as in the word 'pronunciation'. Also, increased salivation makes words sound unclear...

pro-
nun-
ci-

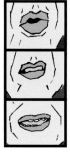

a-
tion

A difficulty in holding onto my thoughts.

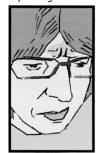

FOR EXAMPLE: EXPRESSING THE FOLLOWING IDEA WHEN I'M DOWN WOULD CAUSE ME DIFFICULTY....

'I would say that my inability to hold thoughts and ideas is the same as my inability to carry objects. I can only do one thing at a time.'

In this situation my speech tends to be punctuated with stuttered pauses as I try to maintain a train of thought. Some people finish my words and sentences for me. I wish they wouldn't because they may not understand what I am trying to say and also they make me feel inadequate.

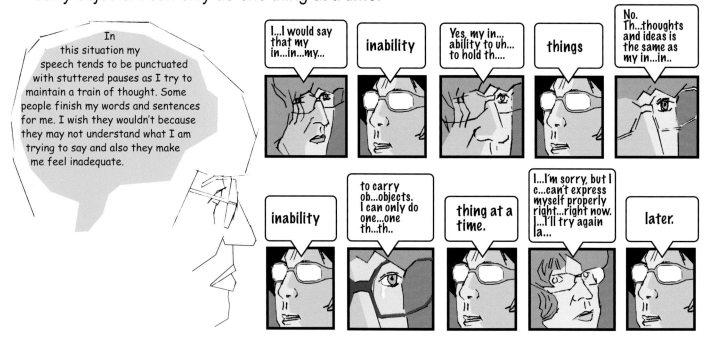

I...I would say that my in...in...my...

inability

Yes, my in... ability to uh... to hold th.....

things

No. Th...thoughts and ideas is the same as my in...in..

inability

to carry ob...objects. I can only do one...one th...th..

thing at a time.

I...I'm sorry, but I c...can't express myself properly right...right now. ...I'll try again la...

later.

ALTHOUGH IT MAY SEEM PECULIAR, I SEE A LINK BETWEEN MY DETERIORATING SPOKEN THOUGHT PROCESSES AND MY DETERIORATING MOVEMENT. JUST AS I BUMP INTO DOORWAYS, LURCH AND VEER OFF COURSE WHEN ATTEMPTING TO WALK IN A STRAIGHT LINE, SO I LOSE TRACK OF THE DIRECTION I AM TAKING IN A CONVERSATION WHEN I TRY TO GIVE AN ACCOUNT OF AN INCIDENT OR ARGUE A POINT. IT COULD BE SAID THAT MY GRIP ON THE SENTENCES I AM TRYING TO GENERATE BECOMES TENUOUS.

THOUGHT

MOTOR

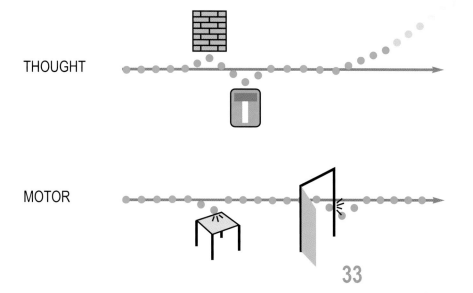

SO, I FEEL THAT PARKINSON'S AFFECTS MY LANGUAGE AND THOUGHT IN A SIMILAR WAY TO ITS EFFECT ON MY MOTOR MOVEMENTS.

33

I ASSUME THAT I SHALL HAVE PARKINSON'S FOR THE REST OF MY LIFE.
SO, IT SEEMS TO ME THAT MY PRESENT SELF SHOULD TAKE ALL POSSIBLE ACTION TO HELP MY FUTURE, LESS CAPABLE SELF.

ONE OF MY CURRENT CONCERNS IS HOW TO PREPARE FOR THE TIME WHEN THE DRUGS BECOME LESS EFFECTIVE. IN TIME I SHALL PROBABLY DEVELOP A TOLERANCE TO THEM. THIS WILL MEAN TAKING MORE AND MORE, MAKING IT LIKELY THAT SEVERE SIDE EFFECTS (DYSKINESIAS AND HALLUCINATIONS) WILL SHOW THEMSELVES.

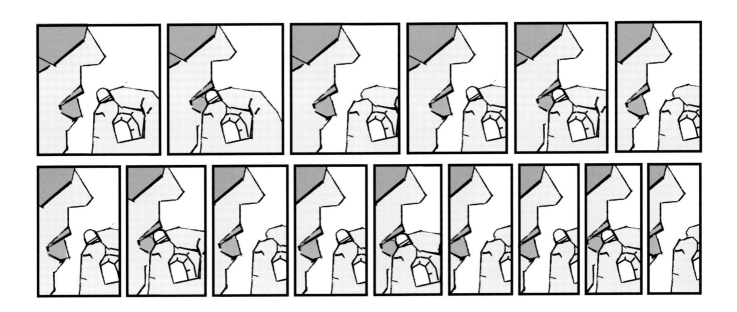

AT PRESENT I HAVE MILD DYSKINESIAS WHICH START IN MY RIGHT FOOT....

AND, WHEN I TALK ENTHUSIASTICALLY, MY FOOT, LEG, ARMS AND HEAD BOB AROUND IN A SORT OF HYPERACTIVE LITTLE DANCE.

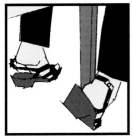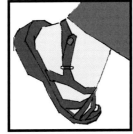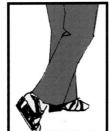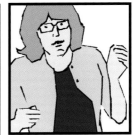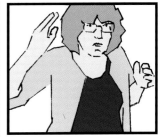

IN THE FUTURE THESE ABNORMAL MOVEMENTS MAY GET A LOT WORSE AND THEY MAY BE ACCOMPANIED BY HALLUCINATIONS.

I AM ALSO CONSIDERING 'DEEP BRAIN STIMULATION' (DBS) WHICH CAN LESSEN TREMORS AND RESULT IN TAKING LESS ANTI-PARKINSON'S DRUGS AND SO, HOPEFULLY AVOID SEVERE SIDE EFFECTS. BUT, IT REQUIRES AN OPERATION.

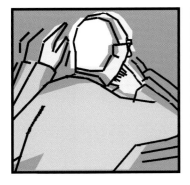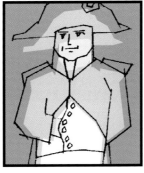

HENCE, AT MY CONSULTANT'S SUGGESTION I AM CONSIDERING THE SELF INJECTION OF APOMORPHINE USING A READY-LOADED DISPOSABLE PEN. APOMORPHINE IS THE STRONGEST OF THE DOPAMINE AGONISTS AND I AM TOLD IT CAN ALLEVIATE OVERPOWERING SYMPTOMS FOR A SHORT TIME (20 MINS TO 1 HOUR).

►

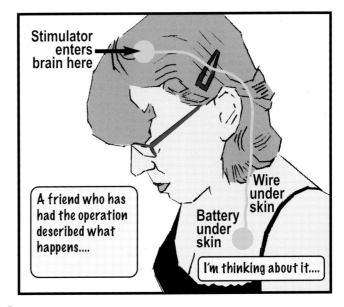

Stimulator enters brain here

Wire under skin

Battery under skin

A friend who has had the operation described what happens....

I'm thinking about it....

I HAVE DESCRIBED THE EXCELLENT EFFECTS OF THE DRUGS I CURRENTLY TAKE~ SINEMET PLUS, ENTACAPONE AND PRAMIPEXOLE.
ALSO, I AM HUGELY ENCOURAGED BY THE AMOUNT OF PARKINSON'S RESEARCH PRESENTLY BEING UNDERTAKEN IN THIS COUNTRY AND ABROAD.

HOWEVER, LOOKING AFTER ONESELF DOES NOT ONLY INVOLVE DRUGS AND OPERATIONS. ALTERNATIVE APPROACHES CAN HELP ONE'S OVERALL SENSE OF WELLBEING AND ENCOURAGE POSITIVITY.

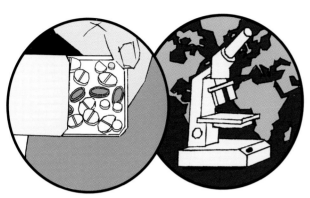

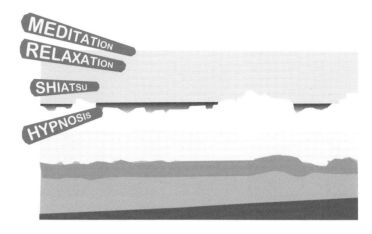

MEDITATION
RELAXATION
SHIATSU
HYPNOSIS

LOOKING AFTER ONESELF ALSO INVOLVES HAVING SUCCESSFUL RELATIONSHIPS WITH OTHER PEOPLE. TO ME THEY ARE CRUCIAL. SO, IN SPITE OF THE DAMAGE PARKINSON'S HAS CAUSED ME, GIVEN THE FOLLOWING SITUATION, I WOULD CHOOSE.....

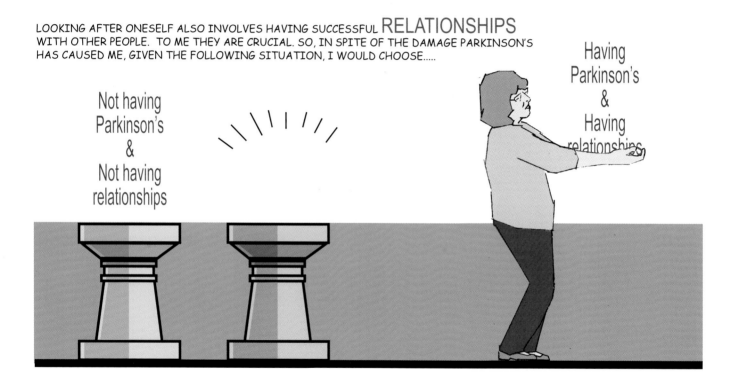

Not having
Parkinson's
&
Not having
relationships

Having
Parkinson's
&
Having
relationships

ABOVE ALL, I BELIEVE IT IS VITAL TO TRY TO UNDERSTAND ONESELF, TO FIND OUT WHAT ONE WANTS TO DO WITH LIFE AND TO ATTEMPT TO ACHIEVE IT.

MY VIEW OF SOME MENTAL SUFFERING, PUT VERY SIMPLY, IS THAT IT OCCURS WHEN A PERSON HAS LOST THE SENSE OF WHO THEY REALLY ARE AND WHAT THEY WANT.

PARKINSON'S HAS HELPED ME REALISE THAT HAVING THIS CONDITION IS LESS IMPORTANT TO ME THAN KNOWING WHO I AM, WHAT I AM DOING, WHAT I AM AIMING FOR AND HOW I RELATE WITH OTHERS.

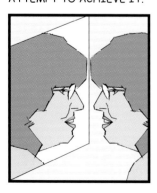

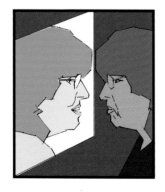

Having
Parkinson's can
cause me to lose
my way for a while
but when all is said
and done it has not
altered my
perception of who
I am and what
I am aiming for
and that is good
enough for me.

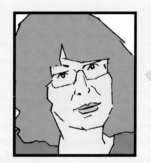

"So, that's my story this far. I have tried to describe my experiences in case they are helpful to others. However, although people with Parkinson's have a lot in common, their experiences can also be very different and what has worked for me, may not work for everyone. Good luck."

Terry

PS. I decided against the brain op.

PPS. Thanks to all the people who
     have given up their seats to me
     on London's buses and underground
     trains over the past ten years.

The company that makes Sinemet has updated
the way in which it produces some of its
tablets. The tablet I have been taking,
Sinemet Plus 25 mg/100 mg (carbidopa 25 mg,
levodopa 100 mg) has changed from a dark
yellow oval tablet (shown in this book) to a
light yellow round tablet.
At the time of going to press I received my
first box of the new tablet.

Old tablet

New tablet